THE RUNNER'S EXPERT GUIDE TO STRETCHING

THE RUNNER'S EXPERT GUIDE TO STRETCHING

Prevent Injury, Build Strength and Enhance Performance

PAUL HOBROUGH

BLOOMSBURY SPORT

LONDON · OXFORD · NEW YORK · NEW DELHI · SYDNEY

BLOOMSBURY SPORT
Bloomsbury Publishing Plc
50 Bedford Square, London, WC1B 3DP, UK

BLOOMSBURY, BLOOMSBURY SPORT and the Diana logo are trademarks of Bloomsbury Publishing Plc

First published in Great Britain 2020

A catalogue record for this book is available from the British Library

Library of Congress Cataloguing-in-Publication data has been applied for

ISBN: PB: 978-1-4729-6532-5; eBook: 978-1-4729-6531-8
2 4 6 8 10 9 7 5 3

Designed by Luana Gobbo
Models' clothing supplied by Saucony®

Printed and bound in Italy by L.E.G.O. S.p.A.

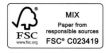

To find out more about our authors and books visit www.bloomsbury.com and sign up for our newsletters

CONTENTS

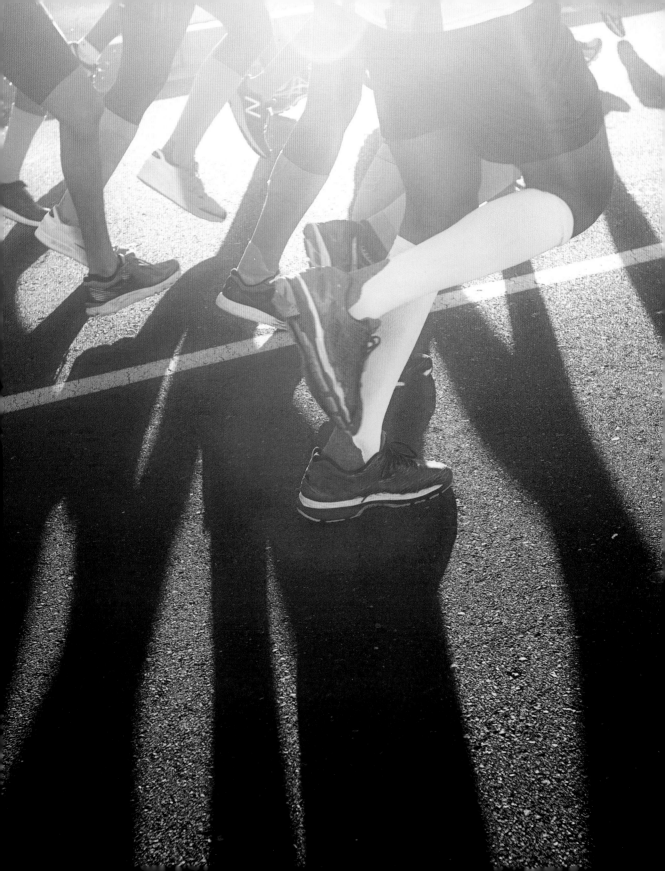

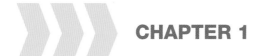

CHAPTER 1

INTRODUCTION

RUNNING. That's what runners do. They run in order to get better at running, right? The more you run, the faster you'll go. Who can argue with that? Well, here I go… If you want to remain injury-free, become a better runner and run faster, I maintain that there's more to training than just running. There, I've said it. And in this book I intend to explain why, and set out what more you need to do to be a fitter, stronger and faster runner.

The misconception that running more miles delivers an improved performance is deep-rooted in the sport. The concept of 'junk miles' – moderate tempo running just to reach a distance goal – has persuaded many runners to incorporate hill runs, speed intervals and form drills into their training, but it is still not uncommon to find even elite athletes diligently turning out 125-mile weeks for no clear reason.

There is no denying the stories of runners who reduce their PBs over a short period of time and these always make a great impression on novice runners. But there is another, less inspiring, side to the stories: the frustrating plateauing and the 30–50 per cent of runners who, over a 12-month period, suffer injuries. These are often written off as inevitabilities – crosses the dedicated runner has to bear – but I aim to show you it doesn't have to be that way.

The simple act of running utilises hundreds of the body's muscles. Every time you run you're using these muscles, forcing them to contract and relax over and over again. Understandably, you might think it's logical that running strengthens muscles: more running equals stronger muscles, meaning fewer injuries and faster times. And the rationale stands up for a while – until a muscle gives way under the strain or fails to develop at the rate necessary to increase speed.

Training is purely a stimulus for your body – a way of making it fight to become fitter, stronger or more flexible. Our body is designed to respond to such stimuli, but a single form of training – in this case, running – will not enable it to deliver beyond its capabilities. If we're going to increase speed and withstand injury, we need to look to other ways to strengthen the parts of the body that deliver the power and bear the load.

WHY WE STRETCH

When physiotherapists and coaches talk about athletes' bodies they will speak of 'range of motion' (ROM), meaning the available amount of movement of a joint, and 'flexibility', meaning the ability of soft tissue structures (such as muscle, tendon and connective tissue) to elongate through the available range of joint motion. Both of these can be vastly improved through stretching. During a stretch, the muscle fibres elongate to their optimum range. The body's nervous system gradually adjusts to the discomfort of the stretch, allowing you to both tolerate and potentially increase the available capacity of the muscle. When we next stretch the muscle, in training or in performance, it should be less likely to become over-stressed, and it will be able to provide more range of movement for the required actions of running.

The range of motion and flexibility required varies across sporting disciplines. Although sportsmen and women all need strong and healthy bodies, a swimmer will have different demands to a cyclist or a footballer. Running has limited requirements compared to, for example, martial arts or gymnastics, and yet there are still many areas of the body key to the running action. Your core muscles keep the spine strong and versatile while providing stability. Your posterior chain – glutes, hamstrings, calves – help propel the body forwards and the shoulders, neck, arms, thighs and feet are almost as critical in the process. The aim of this book is to pinpoint the exercises that specifically target areas of potential weakness or possible strength for the runner.

Few take up running to spend their time exercising indoors, but anyone taking their sport seriously has little alternative: you need to 'train to train'. Just 10–15 minutes a day, or even 30 minutes every other day, spent stretching can build the strength and flexibility of the key muscle areas specific to running. It's time well spent, and can save you weeks of running with a niggling pain – or even months of inactivity while you rehab from injury.

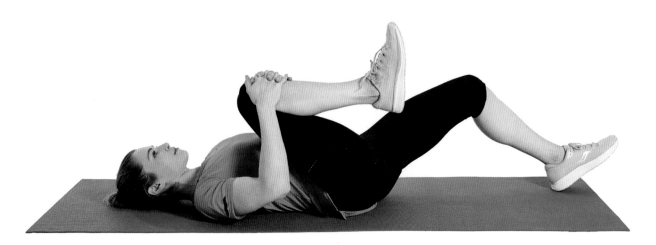

HOW WE STRETCH

Most runners are accustomed to stretching before a run and in a post-run warm-down, but they're often perfunctory, barely remembered warm-ups from gym classes or intuitive stretches based on previous injuries to calves, quads or hamstrings. Far fewer runners practise routines on a daily basis and even those who regularly visit the gym or attend circuit training classes are not performing running-specific exercises.

How we stretch matters. After all, we spend the whole day stretching in some form, from cleaning our teeth to reaching for a can of tomatoes on the top shelf. However, these are not preparing us for sport. There are several methods of stretching that can improve range of motion and enhance muscular performance, and when and why we perform each of them are key to their effectiveness. The ones featured in this book include:

> STATIC STRETCHING – the type with which runners are most familiar, whereby a muscle is slowly stretched to a challenging but comfortable point that is then held for 30–60 seconds.

> DYNAMIC STRETCHING – which involves repeating a movement through a range of motion, such as swinging your leg.

> PASSIVE STRETCHING – where muscles are taken through their range of motion by an external force, such as a strap, your own limbs or with the help of a partner.

Increasingly, experts are favouring the dynamic stretches since they are more effective in building muscle strength, but as the book will detail, there is still an important role for static stretching.

STRENGTH AND CONDITIONING

As a specialist running physiotherapist, I treat elite athletes. They all follow some form of strength and conditioning (S&C) programme and see it as a vital part of their training. Strength and conditioning programmes use prescribed exercises specifically to improve performance in athletic competition. They encompass everything about the physical development of the athlete in regards to their sport, including strength, co-ordination, flexibility, power, agility and balance.

In professional cycling, the idea of 'marginal gains' – incremental improvements from diverse areas that enhance overall performance – has led to some serious advances. In the same way, elite runners are looking for any percentage increase in the strength of key muscles and, for club or casual runners, the benefits can be more than marginal; they can make a significant difference to your strength and, consequently, your running speed and race times.

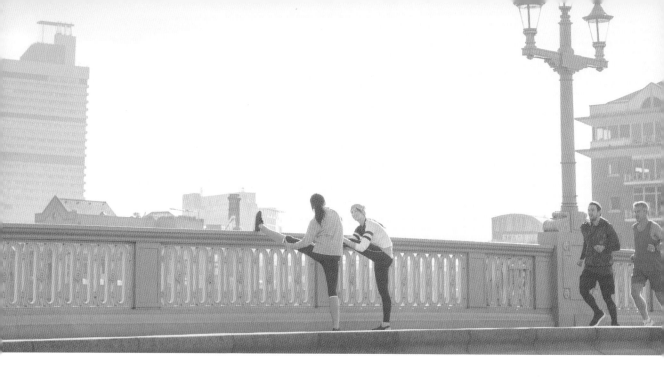

You may already be a gym regular, but if you're doing an exercise and cannot immediately say why you are doing it and what its purpose is for your development, then you are merely weight training. It is imperative for your S&C programme to be relevant not only to you as a runner, but to you as a person, taking into consideration your physical strengths and weaknesses.

HOW TO USE THIS BOOK

You may have already noticed that the book is not just an illustrated series of stretches. It is not intended as a pick 'n' mix of generally beneficial exercises to dip into as you choose. It begins with some science: an explanation of what is happening to your muscles as you run and as you exercise. I need you to understand why you need to do particular stretches; why you are likely to become injured more frequently without them; and why, if you continue to do what you have always done, you will always get what you always got – the plateaus and the injuries.

The self-diagnosis element of the book is essential if you are to use the exercises to improve performance and maximise injury prevention. It will guide you through a series of tests and measures that will enable you to assess your own body and determine a programme that is specific to your requirements and adaptable as you progress. It will help you to identify and avoid potential injuries and explain how to deal with any issues that do arise.

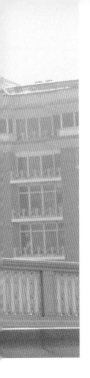

The book divides exercises into beginner, intermediate and advanced levels, but when I use those terms I'm not referring to your running ability. It is not about how fast or how many times a week you run but about your commitment to looking after your body. So, not only does the book allow you to select routines suitable for the level you're currently at, but it also enables you to practise new exercises as you progress.

The stretches and strength training described in this book are fairly comprehensive. There are general exercises that will provide an effective warm-up and cool-down for your run, and a number of stretches and exercises targeting each area of the body. These enable you to build a regular routine customised to your needs, but will also provide you with enough variety to avoid the boredom of repetition.

The final section focuses on improving your performance. The exercises relate to building strength in those areas of the body required to power your run. Again, some of these will be more relevant to you than others, depending on your posture, your physical strengths and weaknesses, and what distance you intend to specialise in.

I enjoyed the response to my first book, *Running Free of Injuries*, especially from those runners who had used it to combat and alleviate pain. In many ways, this is a prequel to that book, because it's the text that every runner should reach for when they're *not* injured. It gives access to a bespoke strength and conditioning programme for every runner, from novice to elite, because every runner needs to stay free of injury and every runner – even those who won't admit it – wants to go faster.

DO THE BASICS WELL

Many runners told me that the main reason they enjoyed *Running Free of Injuries* was that a subject they had previously found challenging had become accessible, jargon-free and even enjoyable. When I talk about things being simple, what I'm trying to get across is that my greatest desire is to get every runner doing the exercises that, while seeming basic, will have the most significant impact on their running. And I want them doing those exercises well. So my aim in this book is to respond and build on that feedback, and provide a wealth of exercises that any runner can practise, at home or in the gym. I'll come back to this idea, but it needs reiterating here – if you want to improve your running performance, prevent injury and enjoy a long-term future as a runner, there's one simple rule: do the basics well.

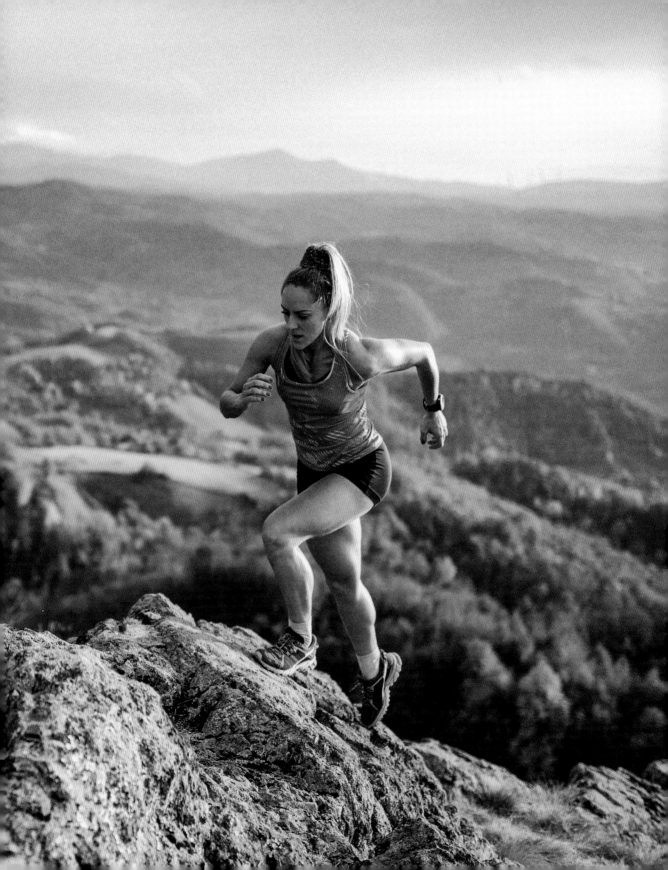

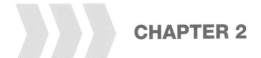

CHAPTER 2

RUNNING EXPLAINED

We all run the same way and we all run differently. The simplicity of running is what attracts so many to the sport, and yet if you look at any parkrun or marathon, you will see hundreds of different types of runner. There are those who glide elegantly along and then there are the shufflers, the striders, the hunchbacks and the arm-swingers (and that strange fella who appears to skip every couple of yards). Who's doing it right? Well, the finer details of perfect running form are keenly debated, but your running style certainly shouldn't be causing you discomfort or injury, and should allow you to increase your speed.

There are basically three ways in which humans move forwards: walking, running and sprinting. We're all pretty familiar with walking – and it doesn't demand a huge amount of the body, using forces of roughly 1.5 times your body weight. Running is a 'spring-driven' movement utilising the elasticity and ability of the Achilles and other tendons to recycle impact energy – for example, the knee is slightly flexed and requires a lot of effort from the muscles to support the joint while the foot is on the ground (and the force is roughly 2–3 times your body weight). Sprinting uses intense anaerobic energy and is a running style adapted for short-term power.

As a runner, you are expecting more of your body than a casual walker. It is required to pivot smoothly, to recycle energy explosively, and sustain repetitive and heavy impact (runners hit the ground with a load of 2.5 times their body weight). It is hardly surprising that over a year up to 50 per cent of runners suffer injuries, with knees, calves, hamstrings, ankles and backs being among the most common, and recurring, problems.

Biomechanics is the science of what causes your body to move forwards. You are propelled by momentum, gravity and the force provided by muscles in your lower body, but much of the work your body does is to keep you stable and balanced. Every time your foot strikes the ground you are landing and then briefly balancing on one leg, but as soon as your foot has reached a stable position, it is then lifted and replaced by the other leg. It is the choices we make within these simple movements – our posture, stride length, cadence and how our foot lands – that determine how much stress is placed on our various joints and muscles, and how efficiently they are used.

The body also makes subconscious decisions. Often called a 'lost sixth sense', proprioception is the body's ability to sense its movement and position. As much as 70 per cent of the information the brain receives about balance, which is key for any runner, comes not from seeing or hearing, but from receptor nerves in the muscles, joints and the ligaments, especially the feet. That's why we don't have to look at our feet constantly when we are running. However, although it seems completely instinctive, through specific exercises we can enhance our vital proprioception and improve our balance.

When professionals refer to a runner's gait, they are simply describing the pattern of how you move forwards. Gait analysis is sometimes undertaken in running shoe shops, but this is usually concentrated on the action of the foot. True gait analysis, which can be done by filming a runner on a treadmill or outside, takes into consideration speed, stride length, trunk rotation and arm swing in terms of how they relate to mobility, stability, flexibility and strength.

THE GAIT CYCLE

In a gait analysis, a physio examines a runner's gait cycle: the period between one foot hitting the ground and that same foot impacting the ground again. The cycle lasts around a second and is made up of three phases:

1. The ground phase (sometimes known as the stance phase) is when the foot is in contact with the ground, i.e. when one leg takes the whole weight of the body. This constitutes around 60 per cent of the cycle.
2. The aerial phase (or swing phase) is the 40 per cent of the time when the foot is in the air, i.e. it is about positioning, balanced movement and recovery.
3. At either end is the very short float phase when neither foot is on the ground.

Initial contact

Initial contact marks the beginning of the ground phase. It is the moment your leading foot – the heel, midfoot or forefoot, depending on your running style and speed – touches terra firma. The other foot, behind you, is now in the aerial phase. The contact period – think of it as a controlled landing – lasts about 0.15 seconds, until your forefoot is on the ground. This is full impact. Your foot pronates (rolls inwards) and the knee slightly bends to help reduce the stress.

Mid-stance

Your weight now shifts to the outside of your foot and is into the mid-stance phase. The knee continues to flex until the leg is directly under the hips. At this point the leg is taking the whole weight of the body as it passes over it. If you took a freeze-frame photo, you'd see that you are basically standing on one leg. It requires hip and core strength to retain balance and puts stress on the whole of the lower leg and lower back.

The terminal phase

The hip and knee joints now extend as the body readies itself for propulsion. As you push forwards, the heel begins to rise, the muscles on the back of the leg contract and the foot pushes off. The leg has now absorbed as much energy as it can and its ankle, knee and hip all extend (straighten) to push the body up and forwards. This, the terminal phase, ends when the toe of your foot (now behind you) leaves the ground (often referred to as 'toe off').

The aerial phase

Once the foot has left the ground, the leg enters the aerial phase. Although this period is a substantial element of the gait cycle, it is of less importance to the biomechanics as there is no weight being borne through the joints and muscles. The hip and knee flex to bring the foot up and then the knee extends to bring the foot back down as it prepares for initial contact, completing the cycle.

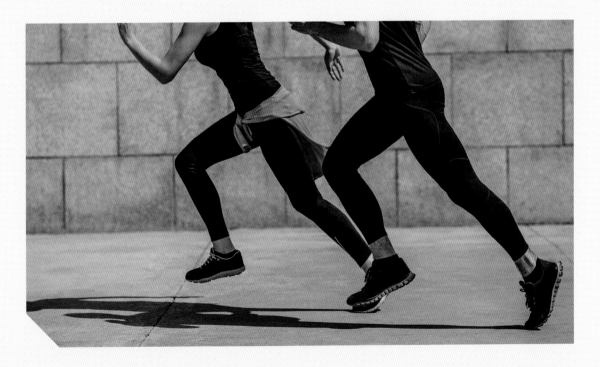

THE LOWER BODY

Through the gait cycle we can see that running is a complex mix of impact, movement, deceleration, energy conversion, limb positioning and balance – most of which is derived from the flexion (bending) and extension (straightening) of muscles and tendons from the hips down. During the gait cycle the body uses hundreds of interconnected muscles and tendons, sometimes the same ones performing different functions. The hips, knees and ankles are points of axis, but the buttocks, thighs, calves and even toes are also key to driving you forwards and keeping you upright and on two legs.

The hip

The role of the hips can't be overstressed. The upper body balances on them and they provide the fulcrum for the leg, which drives our bodies forwards. From the point in mid-stance where your standing foot passes beneath your hips, your leg is extended behind you to push forwards. This is enabled by the buttock 'glutes' – gluteus maximus and gluteus medius – along with the hamstrings behind the knee, contracting to pull the femur (thigh bone) backwards from the hip. Then, as the leg swings forwards before initial contact, it uses the hip flexors at the front of the hip and the rectus femoris (a quadriceps muscle that runs down the thigh). Meanwhile, the muscles of your inner and outer thigh, your adductors and abductors (smaller glute muscles), stabilise your hips and knees.

The knee

The largest joint in the body, the knee primarily absorbs impact and provides stability, although it does generate some power during the terminal phase. Bending and flexing of the knee is the work of the hamstrings, which run down the back of the thigh, and the rectus femoris quadricep, at the front of your thigh, which also helps absorb the impact of landing.

The ankle

The joint nearest to the ground, one ankle takes the full body weight plus the force of gravity in one gait cycle, while playing a crucial role in pushing off the ground. The movement of the ankle is controlled by the calf muscles, including the soleus and the gastrocnemius, via the Achilles tendon (situated at the back of the lower leg), which connects these muscles with the heel. This structure provides stability when the ankle is used as a pivot and creates movement when it is needed to help propel the body.

The foot

The foot is required to absorb the shock of landing and helps the spring forwards into the next stride. A marvellous process called the 'windlass mechanism' sees a whole group of plantar flexor muscles (including the plantaris, which runs from behind the knee to the heel)

convert the supple landing foot into a rigid propulsion foot.
The lifting of the toes (known as dorsiflexion) is provided by the tibialis
anterior, the front part of your shin, which in conjunction with
the perineal muscles on the lateral side tense to spring forwards into
the next stride.

THE UPPER BODY

While the muscles and tendons from your hips down have
been working overtime, it's easy to think that the top half
of your body is just along for the ride. It does, however,
make an invaluable contribution to both stability and
forward thrust and your chest, arms, back and torso are
all vital to balance and effective running.

With each stride of your run, your spine tries to rotate
along with the forward movement of one leg, but it is
your core muscles that keep the body stable. These
muscle sets, which include the rectus abdominus,
obliques, erector spinae and transverse abdominus, are
generally situated around the belly and in the mid- and
lower back, with the glutes, shoulders, neck and hips
providing extra support.

The swing of your arms also counteracts the swivel of
your spine, because your arms work in direct opposition
to the leg, the left arm coming forwards with the drive of
the right leg and vice versa. Your arm action also provides
balance, helps create a rhythm and adds forward propulsion
with the thrust provided by the deltoid muscles in the front of
your shoulder and the latissimus dorsi in your back. As your
body weight is transferred from leg to leg, upper arm biceps and
abdominals are also used to support, co-ordinate and direct the
propulsion, while offering counterbalance and stability.

RUNNING STYLES

With this many elements of the body involved in running, it is
hardly surprising that there are so many different running styles on
display at your local parkrun. Some people are forced to adapt their
natural style because they are carrying injuries or compensating
for previous injuries; other people's styles have been adapted by

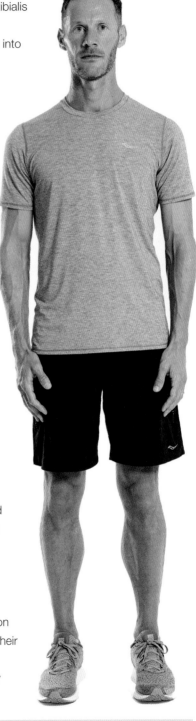

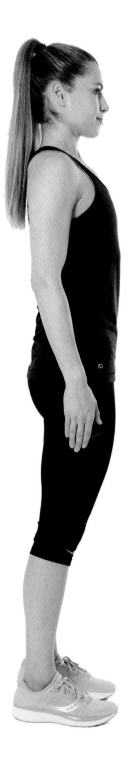

their experience of coaching or according to (factual or mythical) information; and some people simply choose to run like that. Running is just running if you occasionally have to dash for the bus or you have a kick-around with the kids in the garden at the weekend. However, if you are running for 40 minutes or more every week, how you run can affect your physical condition and your ability as a runner.

POSTURE

Good posture begins with the head. Your head should be straight with your eyes focused on the ground 6–7m (20–23ft) ahead of you, with your chin parallel to the ground. This should lead to a straight and aligned neck and back. Your shoulders need to be relaxed and level and your arms should swing backwards and forwards beside your body, not across your body.

If your head and shoulders are in the right position then your upper body should follow, taking an upright position with a straight back. Coaches often refer to 'running tall', which is a good description as long as you don't take it to mean being stiff. If your spine is too rigid, it will lose its ability to absorb stress and there will be more impact on the knees, hamstrings and glutes.

Finally, the hips are your centre of gravity and all being well, they will remain level as the pelvis rotates with each stride. The danger for fatigued runners or those with a weak core is that the pelvis tilts forwards and pushes the hips back. This affects the hamstrings and glutes, and can cause back and hip problems. Equally debilitating is the Trendelenburg gait. Caused by weakness and poor muscle control in the lower body, it leads to one hip dropping lower than the other, which can cause muscles from the calf to the shoulder to compensate.

CADENCE AND STRIDE

Your speed depends on your cadence (steps per minute) and the length of your stride. The average recreational runner usually takes around 150 to 170 steps per minute, whereas elite runners are running at nearer the 200 mark.

Stride length is the distance from the toe of one foot to the toe of the other foot when you are in motion. Stride lengths vary with the height of the runner. A suitable stride length finds your feet landing directly underneath your body with the knee slightly flexed on impact. Overstriding, which is a common problem in runners, occurs when your lower leg extends out in front of your body. The longer the stride, the higher you jump in the air and the greater the impact on landing. This also leads to a straighter knee, reducing shock absorbency.

You can run faster by speeding up your steps (also known as your cadence) or by taking longer strides. If you're seeking to run faster, look at increasing your cadence before your stride length, because increasing the length of your strides depends on your physical condition, with hip flexibility and glute strength being the key factors in taking longer forward strides.

PRONATION AND SUPINATION

Pronation is where the foot naturally rolls inwards towards the medial longitudinal arch as we walk or run (for heel strikers) and supination is the opposite, where the foot remains in a more lateral position along the little toe side of the foot. Let's clear something up first of all: neither is bad. There has been a sense over the last 20 years that over-pronation was a terrible affliction that led to many an injury, but this is not the case. The way your foot falls naturally is not something that you necessarily need to block or change, but you do need adequate strength and gradual loading of your training to allow your musculo-skeletal system to accept the force and the duration of your runs.

That being said, if you are becoming injured over and over again, have tried all of the exercises contained within this book and are unable to continue with your training due to dysfunction and pain, then it may well benefit you to have a bespoke orthotic created for your foot by a podiatrist. Orthotics fit inside your shoe and essentially remove the burden from overworked muscles. They can also slow down the movements of pronation or supination, or even just change when these occur durng the gait cycle. An orthotic is a prescription, much as you would need a prescription for poor eyesight, but orthotics can also serve as a form of treatment. I would prescribe an orthotic for a runner once every other stone had been overturned in terms of strength, flexibility and technical advancement. I have at times used orthotics as a temporary measure as they can help faster than a muscle group can strengthen, providing a window of opportunity for an athlete to run with less pain, thus allowing more time for their strength and conditioning (S&C) to catch up – whereupon the devices can be removed. For some runners they are a life sentence and will need renewing approximately every two years.

FOOT CONTACT

You can be a rearfoot, midfoot or forefoot runner depending on how your foot hits the ground as it lands. Around 80 per cent of recreational runners are rearfoot runners, or heel strikers. Midfoot evangelists argue that the nearer the heel you land, the greater the impact on the knee. There is some truth in this, but in general your body will adapt to the forces you place on it regularly, unless there is major dysfunction – in which case this will be exacerbated and may result in injury. It is fairly well established that forefoot strikers load the Achilles whereas heel strikers are more prone to loading the knee. It doesn't follow, however, that you are likely to create injury in these areas if you are one or the other, it simply means as a forefoot striker you should work on the calf strength and Achilles pre-hab and heel strikers should work to protect the knee. It also doesn't follow that if you are a mid-foot runner you are better off – you are betwixt and between, which doesn't make you a better or a worse runner.

Forefoot running is widely accepted as being faster. Sprinters land on the fronts of their feet, but while many elite distance runners also appear to land on their forefoot, slow camera footage can often betray a minuscule heel-strike. A study was able to show that 80 per cent of elite runners were natural supinators and therefore more likely to forefoot strike, whereas 80 per cent of recreational and club runners had a pronating foot and so would naturally heel-strike. Pervading forefoot evangelism means that many of those who would naturally heel-strike try a forefoot stance, and while this may assist them, conversely, it may betray their natural style. The core message is that you should stick to what you feel comfortable doing because changing your habitual style can also increase your injury risk. You may well be better off running in your lifelong, learned style and working harder on your S&C programme. However, do be *aware* of how you land, because you need to recognise where the stress is impacting in your body and be prepared to strengthen the relevant areas. Also, be aware that your strike position can change as you run: if you are sprinting for the line, you might change from heel strike to forefoot.

A targeted strength and conditioning programme will allow you to adapt your own natural style and also make you faster. If all the runners attempting the onerous change of style gave that same commitment to S&C, foot contact might become a moot point.

HYPERMOBILITY AND HYPOMOBILITY

There are a myriad of conditions you might face as a runner and here I am simply mentioning the two extremes of a flexibility spectrum, which may occur naturally in some of you. Hypermobility is a condition which makes joints extra-flexible due to a reduced amount of collagen in the connective tissue. Hypomobility is the opposite, an unusually large amount of collagen in the connective tissue, often meaning stretching elicits little short-term benefit and touching your toes is something that other people do.

For those with hypomobility, stretch all you can. It may not be comfortable but at least try to gain a few per cent extra in your range of movement. Stick at it for life, even join a yoga class, and accept you might be the only person who needs a pulley rope to cut your toenails.

However, if you are hypermobile (like my daughter) then you will find stretching very easy and probably have a party trick to hand where you place your feet behind your head, or can put your toe in your mouth (gross, I know – but I've seen it done). Take a qualified fitness professional's advice, but I would suggest that if you are hypomobile then a commitment to foam rolling your muscles and using the strength exercises in this book will serve you much better than performing the stretches. Hypermobility, by its very definition, means you are probably a little 'too flexible' so you may well be advised to avoid stretching altogether, to keep your soft tissues (including tendons and ligaments) as tight as possible.

FOOTWEAR

Shoe manufacturers have gone through a full 180-degree pivot in the last 10 years or more. For a while, everyone was opting for shoes with various gradients of medial support to 'remove' pronation, which today sounds completely crazy. Pronation is a natural physiological movement necessary for foot mechanics and load acceptance. These shoes became heavier and heavier and probably caused more injuries than they resolved. Then in the blink of an eye, the fashion changed to minimalist footwear. This reversal created a dramatic upturn in revenue for physiotherapists like me. In fact, many manufacturers had silently reduced the heel-to-toe drop of a shoe from in excess of 12 degrees down to between 4–8 degrees overnight. The effect was huge and, sadly for all the runners, meant my diary was full to bursting with lower-limb complaints. It started the trend for healthcare professionals to suddenly advertise themselves as 'running specialists'.

The fact remains that you are an individual and in many ways your foot shape and type are as individual as your fingerprint. Your running technique has been created over time, from a mix of how running felt when you were a child through to emulating your favourite sports person as you watched them move. Either way, you have unknowingly honed this skill over the years and it's now yours. No pair of shoes can have the same impact as a great coach, who knows how to make some micro adjustments over a protracted time period that will benefit your technique rather than totally rewrite it.

There are also other factors that you need to take into consideration, including:

❱ TERRAIN: If you are mainly running on roads and paths you might think about choosing a shoe with an element of cushioning to soften the repeated impact. Off-road running, on the other hand, often makes tread a key factor in providing traction on slippery surfaces.

❱ STRIKE POINT: If you are a heel striker, some additional cushioning in that area could provide extra comfort and minimise impact injury.

❱ DISTANCE: Among those running a half-marathon or above, a degree of support and cushioning is often of some consolation in the latter stages of a run.

❱ WEIGHT: If you weigh 80kg (13 stone) or more you are putting considerable strain on your ankles and feet, so it makes sense to ensure your footwear offers some support and cushioning.

❱ COMFORT: This is perhaps the most important consideration of all. Make sure you feel right in the shoes. Try them on in the shop, if possible running on a treadmill. Don't get too tight a fit as your feet will swell as you run and allow 1cm (½in) of extra space in the toe for natural slide.

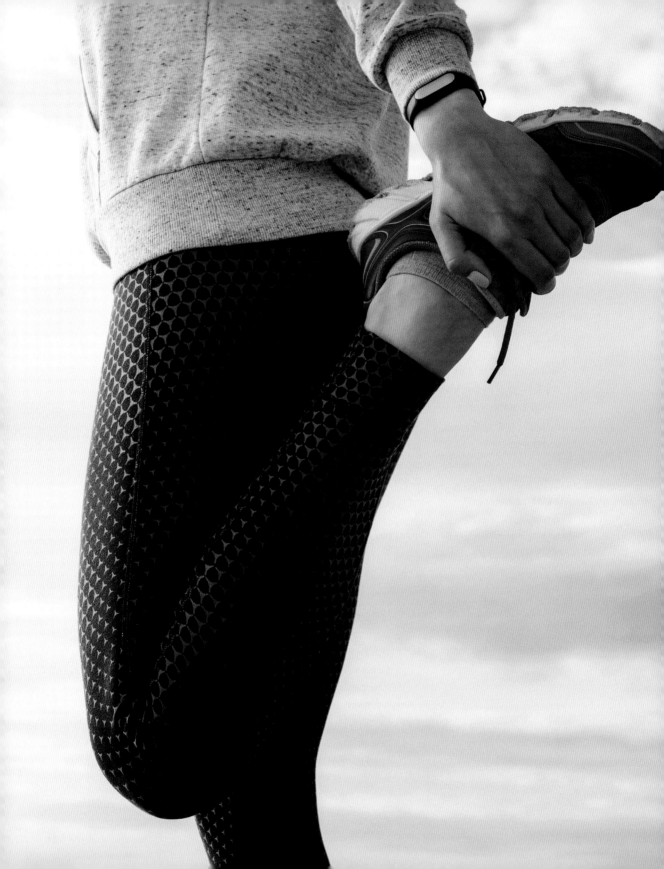

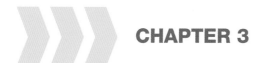

CHAPTER 3

STRETCHING

What's in a good stretch? It can feel good when you get up in the morning and have a good yawn, pushing your arms out to welcome the day. Or, it can feel slightly painful when you're desperately reaching up to the top shelf for a can of beans. It's just a matter of degree. Stretching is simply extending a muscle beyond its customary range of motion (ROM), which is determined by what that muscle does and how flexible it is – how far we can reach, bend or turn.

Stretching, as it will be described in this book, is the process of placing limbs in a particular position that will optimise the available length of the muscle and associated soft tissues. There are many benefits to stretching, including reducing tension in the muscles, enhancing muscular co-ordination and increasing blood circulation around the body, but its capacity to increase the ROM in the joints is central to our conditioning as runners.

Stretching is centred around the muscles as they are the most important factor in ROM. Bones and joints have some impact on flexibility, but there is little we can do to affect them, whereas ligaments, tendons, skin and scar tissue do also react to the stretching process. The crucial factor for achieving a greater ROM is the elongation of the muscle and connective tissue. Each muscle fibre is made up of lots of cell sections called sarcomeres. The aim of stretching is to release any tension in each of these segments of muscle.

The science explaining what is happening in your body when you stretch is complex, with some areas still a matter of debate by experts. For our requirements, just some basic facts will suffice. By stretching, we are developing the relationship between our muscles and our nervous system. Nerve endings are dispersed throughout the muscle and tendon. When the muscle is put under stress, it is these nerves that sound the alarm through discomfort, pain and resistance. By stretching, we are reassuring the nervous system that it can tolerate a greater degree of muscle extension without having to fire off these signals.

Through a regular stretching routine a number of other changes can be induced within the muscles and associated tissues. Muscular tension is reduced and the efficiency of your muscles increases, allowing the same extension to be repeated with less energy. The blood flow to your muscles is also increased, maximising the supply of essential nutrients and decreasing the build-up of lactic acid (waste product), which causes soreness and fatigue in the muscles.

As we saw in the previous chapter, a plethora of muscles are at work in the process of running, with a series of joints flexing and extending. Flexibility is a vital element in reducing the chances of injury and improving performance, and the easiest way to improve flexibility is by stretching the relevant and vulnerable muscles used.

WAYS TO MOVE

There are a number of ways of stretching safely, each with their own benefits and effectiveness and suited to different situations and goals. The various forms of stretches can basically be divided into two groups, dynamic and static, which are undertaken with or without movement, respectively.

Dynamic stretching

Dynamic stretching is characterised by movement accompanying the stretch. It involves controlled, gentle movements of joints and muscles through a full range of motion, often mimicking the actions they undertake in a particular sport or activity. They facilitate an active tightening of muscles as well as helping to increase muscle temperature and decrease muscle stiffness. Examples of dynamic stretches include a repeated swinging of the arm or high knee marching. They are relatively safe as muscles are moved within their range of motion without running the risk of being injured or torn, which makes them perfect for a warm-up before running.

Ballistic stretching

This is a form of dynamic stretching utilised by gymnasts, dancers and some elite athletes where it is required for their sport. Ballistic stretching uses the momentum of a moving body part or a limb in an attempt to encourage it beyond its normal available range of motion. Due to the high injury risk associated with this form of stretching, it is not advised for runners.

Static stretching

Static stretching is what many people commonly perceive stretching to be: extending the muscle to a point at which there is a slight discomfort, then holding it for a short period of time, usually around 30–60 seconds. When performed correctly, static stretches are relatively safe and can improve your flexibility. An example of a static stretch is the hamstring stretches you'll find on pp. 139–141.

Passive stretching

This is a form of static stretching that involves you placing your body in a position that you don't have to work to hold. This could involve something as simple as a wall or the floor but often requires you to use a hand, a partner or a piece of apparatus, such as an exercise ball, to hold a position. Passive stretching is considered a very safe way of increasing suppleness as it does not involve abrupt movements and is unlikely to make someone exceed their muscles' limits.

PNF (Proprioceptive Neuromuscular Facilitation)

This uses both passive stretching and isometric exercise (*see* p. 39). PNF follows a pattern of a 10-second stretch to the point of discomfort, a five- to 10-second isometric contraction and 30-second stretch slightly beyond the range of your first stretch. PNF stretches use the sudden relaxing of the muscle to allow the nervous system to become familiar with the increased muscle length exerted by the final passive stretch. This combination of extension and contraction of muscles is excellent for improving range of motion, targeting specific muscle groups and re-aligning muscle fibres and connective tissue (important after a heavy workout). It is an advanced technique that is often performed inappropriately. With this in mind, it would be best to seek the advice of a qualified physio to optimise the use of this in your training.

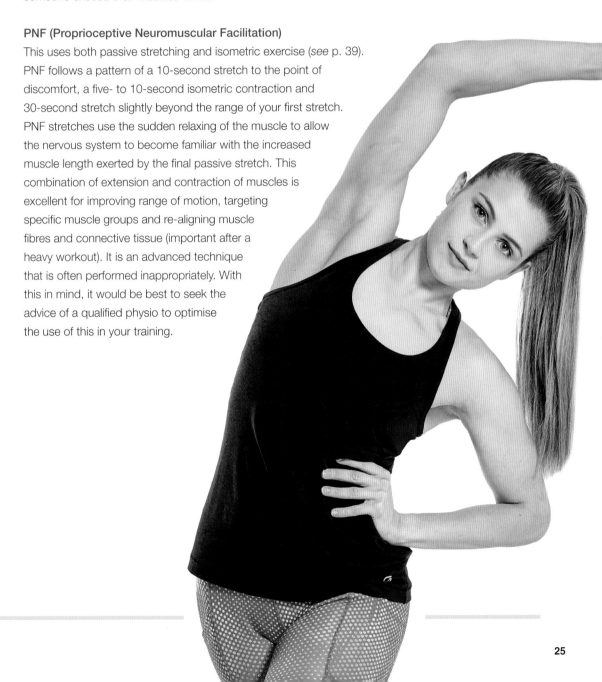

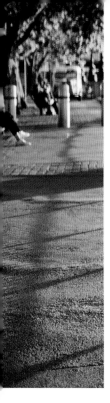
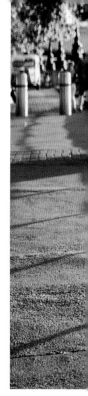

CHOOSING THE RIGHT TYPE OF STRETCH

The warm-up

Since the beginning of the 21st century it has been pretty much universally accepted that any warm-up should begin with a series of dynamic stretches. These kinds of exercises should be fluid, continual and undertaken with care and might include brisk walking, light lunging, high kicks and backwards butt kicks and knee lifts. They should be undertaken before any run or workout.

Light stretching with movement raises the temperature of the muscles and improves the blood circulation. By imitating the movements used in running, you prepare the muscles to be used by bringing them close to, but not exceeding, the ROM that will be required. Dynamic stretching also prepares your whole body for exercise, warming those muscles that are required to work together or provide support as well as focusing your balance and co-ordination before you begin more strenuous activity.

Static stretches should not form part of your warm-up until the dynamic stretches have been completed. Unless there are specific tight muscle areas that need attention, there is little to be gained from static stretching at this stage and there is an increased risk of damaging muscles before they are warm. Some studies even conclude that passive stretching before activity can impair performance by putting too much strain on key muscle areas and reducing strength.

Mid-activity

No one wants to interrupt a run and spend valuable minutes stretching, but there are occasions – especially in long-distance running events such as marathons – when this may be necessary in order for the runner to continue. Certain easy and targeted static, active stretches or even massages can be performed at the side of the track and may provide a considerable easing of pain. This technique is often employed by athletes carrying a niggle through a marathon event, which while not ideal, is very common.

Warm-down

A five- to 10-minute cooling-down period after a workout or run allows for a gradual recovery of pre-exercise heart rate and blood pressure. This aids the removal of lactic acid from your muscles, which lessens the likelihood of cramping or muscle spasm. A short, gentle session of dynamic stretching that decreases in intensity should be followed by static stretching to ease muscles which have shortened during the activity. Stretching helps these muscles re-establish their resting length and reduces the chances of stiffness and injury.

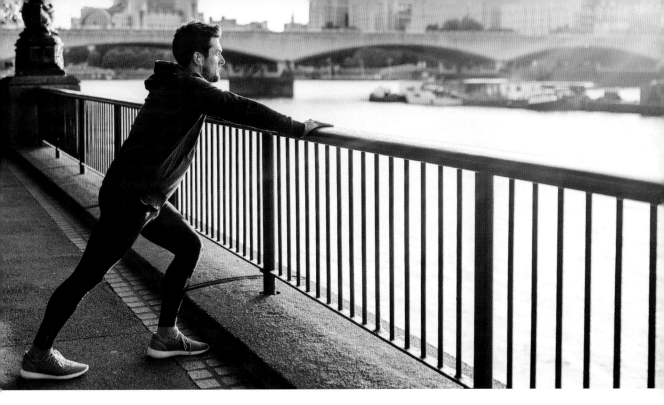

STRENGTH AND CONDITIONING

Although runners require a general level of flexibility across the body, their training needs to include S&C work that is targeted to the activity. A regular general workout in the gym might make you fit, but it won't necessarily make you a better runner: you may build heavy muscles in areas not required for running, or reach a level of flexibility that causes instability in key joints when on the move. The sport places serious demands on specific muscle areas and any exercises need to be considered and directed.

While most popular forms of stretches obviously fall within the realm of static stretching, we can be more precise and look at passive and PNF exercises. Active stretching maintains joint flexibility, but it is the more strenuous stretches that have an effect on ROM.

INJURY

On suffering anything more than slight muscular pain, the first reaction should be to stop, or reduce as much as possible, any activity that puts stress in that area. If it is severe or does not respond to rest, it is advisable to see a physiotherapist before attempting any stretches. When it is a slight niggle, or under a prescribed programme from the physio, a combination of dynamic and static stretches will most likely be a part of your rehabilitation plan, alongside strengthening exercises.

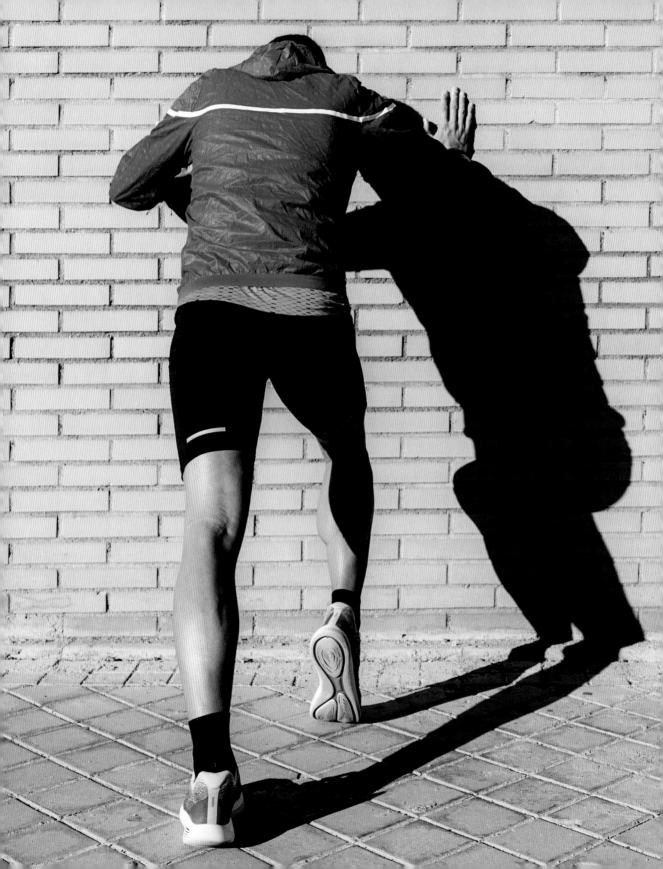

CHAPTER 4

MUSCLE MYTHS: STRETCHING SCIENCE DEBUNKED

Physiotherapy is a fast-changing world. Attitudes to stretching have changed radically over the past 50 years and continue to be adapted as new theories emerge year on year. Physios have a professional responsibility to keep abreast of changes, but it is more difficult for club and recreational runners, who may find it is all too easy to pick up out-dated or even ill-founded information. So it seems worthwhile to look at a few of the common truisms of stretching and see how much scientific truth they hold.

》 MYTH: STRETCHING BEFORE RUNNING REDUCES YOUR PERFORMANCE
There is no evidence that dynamic stretches in a warm-up will affect performance adversely, but it certainly has some positive psychological and physical impact – preparing the mind and body for activity – and some studies have indicated that it may even provide a small boost in power. However, in regards to static stretching, the opposite is true. Static stretching will not aid performance. In fact, it can have a negative effect on muscle strength, power and endurance.

》 MYTH: YOU DON'T NEED TO STRETCH BEFORE A RUN, ONLY AFTERWARDS
As laid out in the previous chapter, a warm-up of dynamic stretches is advisable before any run. As there is sufficient scientific evidence to suggest it can help in preventing injury as well as getting you 'in the zone', the strongest argument is surely, why not? The misconception is probably founded in the lack of benefit in static stretching before activity. However, post-run, there are some arguments for the effectiveness of both dynamic and static exercises in preventing soreness in joints and muscles.

MYTH: STRETCHING CAN CAUSE INJURY

Both dynamic and passive stretching should be perfectly safe activities if performed correctly and with due care and caution. Stretching should never be painful. Where injuries do occur they are generally due to poor body positioning, stretching an injured or cold muscle, or stretching being performed with too much vigour.

MYTH: THE FASTEST GUY AT OUR RUNNING CLUB HASN'T EVER STRETCHED OR EVER BEEN INJURED – SO NOW I DON'T STRETCH ANYMORE

Some runners are born lucky, others have to make their own luck through S&C work and sensible preparation. Everyone will also have a different collagen density (*see* p. 20), meaning some people need to stretch more than others. When it comes to running, we are not born equal; some are more injury-prone than others and once you get one injury, especially if it's mismanaged, more injuries often follow. Equally, stretching can't guarantee you won't pick up an injury, but it can reduce the chances and facilitate a faster recovery.

MYTH: YOU CAN OVERSTRETCH

Overstretching is possible, but it's not a frequently encountered problem and is reasonably easy to avoid. It can arise if you have not warmed up sufficiently or are not focused on the exercise and stretching with care. Overstretching typically occurs when a muscle or joint is pushed well beyond its normal range of motion – for example, reaching for a squash shot or similar – and can create problems such as strains, inflammation or tears in muscle tissue. Overstretching can be avoided by performing careful, controlled and gradual stretches. Stop when you begin to feel tightness in the muscle and a very slight discomfort and do not continue to the point that you feel pain.

MYTH: YOU ONLY NEED TO STRETCH ON RUNNING DAYS

Pre- and post-run stretches might be good preparation and ward off some stiffness, but in order for strength and conditioning training to pay off, it requires some level of commitment. If you are looking to improve your performance you should be looking to do 30-minute workouts two or three times a week. Workouts are best performed on days following runs and neither activity should lead to underperformance in the other. It is also essential that rest days are incorporated in the schedule as your muscles need time to repair themselves and this is when the strengthening actually takes place. Yes, elite runners train twice per day, but they have spent years building up to this and avoid back-to-back sessions.

❱ MYTH: STRENGTH TRAINING WILL MAKE ME BULK UP

The aim of strength training is to make muscles stronger, not always bigger. Your muscles might be toned but not bodybuilder massive. There are two basic reasons for this. First, you will be performing low-resistance exercises rather than lifting the extreme weights needed to bulk up. Second, you are a runner – a sport that counteracts the muscle-building effect. Bodybuilders don't run, they eat specifically to fuel muscle growth, whereas you are using that energy to fuel your runs.

❱ MYTH: FOAM ROLLING IS EASIER THAN STRETCHING AND IT PROVIDES THE SAME BENEFITS

Foam rolling – self-massage using a lightweight, cylindrical tube of compressed foam – is used to target areas of muscular tension. It is great for treating small tight spots and knots. The benefits of stretching and foam rolling do overlap, but in most of us only stretching will aid and increase ROM and flexibility. However, those with hypermobile joints may be well advised to use a foam roller to assist their muscles instead of stretching.

❱ MYTH: I GO TO YOGA CLASSES SO I DON'T NEED A STRETCHING PROGRAMME

It is easy to see why yoga might be viewed as a great match for runners: it employs gentle stretches that improve flexibility, and positions that are suitably challenging to also strengthen. It is a great accompaniment for those who run for overall fitness. However, for those who are looking to improve their run times, general yoga classes may not provide sufficient specific stretching and/or strengthening. Running S&C focuses on ROM, whereas yoga concentrates on flexibility; the running gait is dependent on energy gained from the elasticity and strength of muscles and this requires targeted strength training as well as general stretching exercises.

❝ Attitudes to stretching have changed radically over the past 50 years ❞

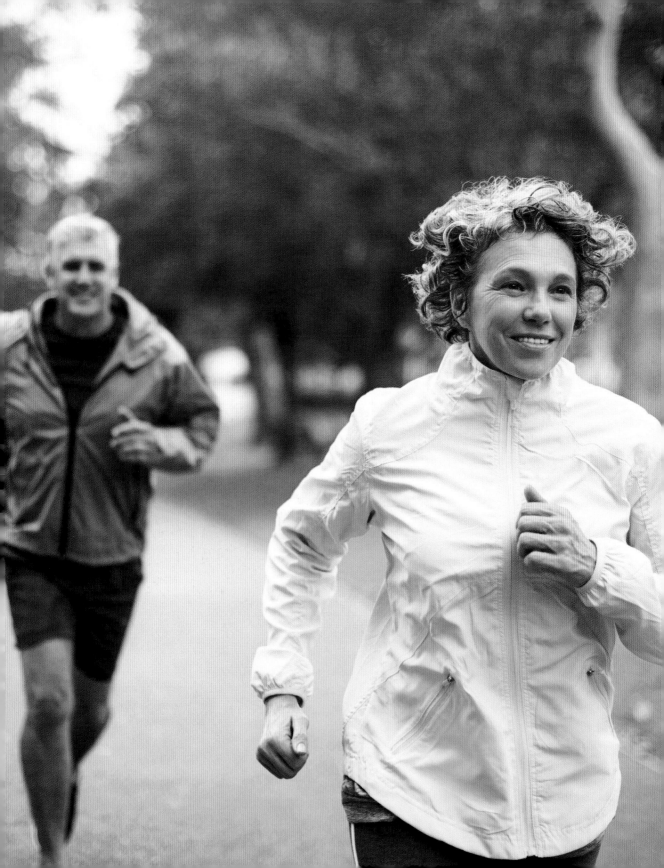

CHAPTER 5

STRENGTH TRAINING

For many years, weight training was seen as counter-productive to runners. Why would you want to bulk up with heavy muscles? Body building and muscle toning seemed a vanity project compared to getting out and putting in some hard miles. However, times and attitudes change. Not all training is the same. Runners realised they were able to strengthen the muscles not to look buff, but to be stronger and faster athletes.

Strength training is a targeted form of exercise that can improve muscle strength, endurance and lean muscle mass. It involves exercises in which muscles are made to work harder than usual. Most movements or support of weighty objects (including the human body) – such as carrying a small child or climbing the stairs – can be considered a form of strength training, but we are interested in specific exercises that focus on a target area, or muscle groups of benefit to the runner.

> "Running relies on many types of muscle strength: power, agility, endurance and explosive strength ... all can be improved through strength training"

MUSCULAR STRENGTH

Muscular strength is defined as the maximal force that a muscle or muscle group can generate during a single bout of exercise (Kenny, Wilmore, & Costil, 2015). It relies on the size of your muscle fibres and the ability of nerves to activate them. The simplest demonstration of muscular strength is weightlifting: when you lift 90kg (200lb) you are exhibiting twice the strength of a 45kg (100lb) lift. However, the tasks we set our muscles in everyday life and in sport are not confined to single movements or to simple actions. Muscle strength can be defined in different terms, including:

❯ POWER: The level of force that can be produced by a muscle or muscle group as explained above.

❯ AGILITY: The ability to change the direction of the body – a combination of balance, speed, strength and co-ordination that requires muscles to operate in a multiplanar environment.

❯ ENDURANCE: The ability to perform a consistent level of muscle force over an extended period of time.

❯ EXPLOSIVE STRENGTH: Producing the maximum amount of force in the minimal amount of time.

WHAT DOES STRENGTH DO FOR A RUNNER?

It is clear, even from such simple definitions, that running relies on many of these strength types. In particular, muscle power is vital in determining the force you can drive into the ground; agility is essential in balance and posture; explosive strength drives your spring; and endurance is necessary to maintain your efficient running action.

The effectiveness of all of these is reliant on a number of characteristics of the body, including the power muscles can exert, the efficiency of the oxygen and nutrient supply, the muscles' resilience in performing repetitive tasks and the ability of nerves to activate muscle fibres – all of which can be improved through strength training.

The strength of a runner's muscles and connective tissues is also a major factor in avoiding injury. Running puts considerable stress on hips, knees and many other joints. It is the strength of these and supporting muscle groups that enables us to endure sustained impact and retain a core balance, which prevents the body from putting undue pressure on vulnerable areas.

RESISTANCE TRAINING

Although many gym weight machines have been specifically designed for strength training, these tend to produce 'stupid' muscles that work in isolation and runners need functional strength. So, this book will explain simple techniques that can be performed with the minimum of apparatus. These are exercises using body weight, such as calf raises, crunches and leg squats, or ones that use easily obtainable equipment, such as resistance bands, exercise balls or free weights.

The effectiveness of all of these exercises is reliant on them being repeated a number of times in one session – they will be explained in terms of 'repetitions' (reps), which is one full completion of a stretch or exercise; 'load', meaning the amount of weight or resistance employed (which is as individual as eye glasses and cannot be prescribed by a book); and 'sets', a group of repetitions done together with minimum rest. So you will be given sets of reps and it is expected that you will take time to experiment with the right load for these parameters.

PROGRESSIVE OVERLOAD

The magic ingredient of strength training is 'progressive overload': making your muscles work ever harder. It is the most important factor in getting results from your training and is based on the simple truth that your body will not change unless it is forced to. In order for a muscle to be strengthened, it must be made to adapt to a tension that exceeds that previously experienced. This can be effected by an incremental increase of repetitions or load, or by decreasing the rest intervals during a set. If you're looking to focus on strength, you may wish to increase the resistance, whereas increased muscle endurance can be better achieved through more reps, with less rest between sets, and less load.

> **"Progressive overload is the most important factor in getting results from your training ... the simple truth is that your body will not change unless it is forced to"**

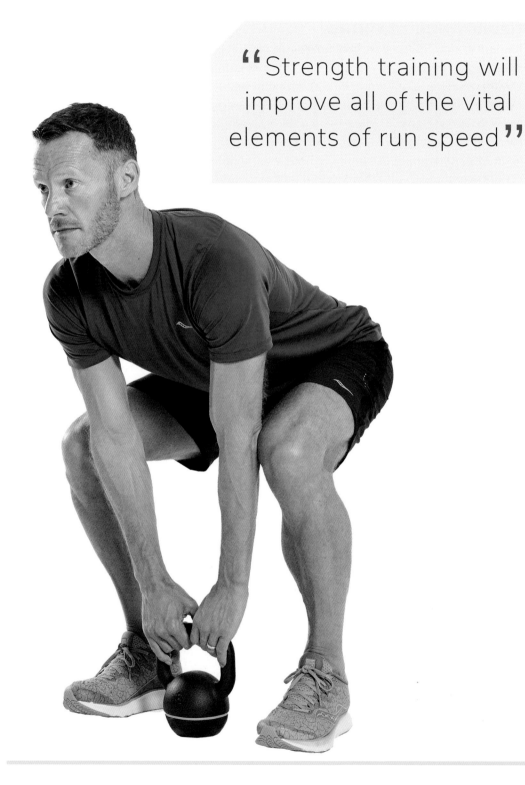

"Strength training will improve all of the vital elements of run speed"

A graded exercise programme will have a latent response lasting at least 36 hours. What this means is that the protein within the muscle needs time to sythesise and repeating the same training within this period may prevent this from happening. Therefore you should try to avoid exercising the same muscle in the same way (for example, high weight, low reps) within this time period. This latent period is one of the reasons why delayed onset muscle soreness (DOMS) is so much worse two days after a heavy session or race rather than the morning after. Runners can train every day, even twice a day, as long as their programme respects this and combines, for example, heavy weight training with a recovery run later that day as opposed to going to the gym again.

STRENGTH TRAINING FOR PERFORMANCE

There is little doubt that for runners with little or no experience of strength training, a programme of stretching and lifting will nearly always deliver improvements in long-term performance. This is because strength training will improve all of the vital elements of a faster run speed. There are several key areas that you are looking to improve through strength training:

- ❯ CORE STRENGTH When you run, your abs and back muscles are tasked with stabilising your upper body. If they are unable to do this effectively, the body compensates with other movements. This leads to an inefficient gait and decreases the power of the push-off.

- ❯ ANAEROBIC POWER This increases the ability of the muscles to work without enough oxygen and when lactic acid is produced. You become more efficient at removing, or at least dealing with, the waste product effectively, meaning you can maintain a higher intensity for longer periods of time.

- ❯ NEUROMUSCULAR EFFICIENCY Developing the nervous system allows better inter-muscular co-ordination of all relevant muscles, leading to greater force.

- ❯ RUNNING ECONOMY An improvement in muscle strength, neurological response and flexibility results in a more efficient use of energy with every step.

- ❯ POWER DEVELOPMENT An increase in explosive strength gives a runner more power, which has many benefits, including a sprint finish.

STRENGTH TRAINING TO PREVENT INJURY

One of the main factors in making progress as a runner is staying fit. Injuries can hamper your run, cause harm in other parts of the body or prevent you from running at all. You might be a strong runner in terms of running 80km (50 miles) a week, but if you don't invest time in strengthening your body, almost certainly you will pay the price somewhere along the line. A bespoke strength training programme cannot guarantee this won't happen but it certainly tilts the odds in your favour. Here are some of the key areas that strength training can benefit:

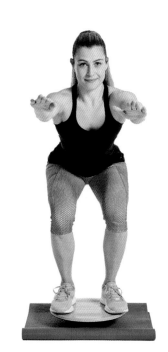

❭ POSTURE Certain imbalances occur naturally in the body, such as left and right knees flexing unequally or some muscles becoming so strong they overpower others. Correcting these imbalances with training can reduce the risk of injury to those joints, ligaments and muscles under stress.

❭ STRUCTURAL FITNESS Strength exercises increase the ability of your bones, ligaments, tendons and muscles to withstand the impact of running. For example, well-developed abs and back muscles result in a strong core that helps protect your spine.

❭ MUSCLE GROUPS By targeting runners' key muscle groups, areas such as the abductors, gluteal muscles, hamstrings, quads and hip flexors can be fortified, reducing the chances of common injuries, including shin splints, plantar fasciitis (the pain in the bottom of your foot, around your heel and arch that is increasingly known as plantar fasciopathy), runner's knee or iliotibial band syndrome (ITBS).

❭ BALANCE A strong core is essential to balance, but so too is proprioception – the body's natural sense of balance. Work on this area can reduce risk of injury through instability, especially for those who run on uneven surfaces.

❭ BONE STRENGTH Running assists bone maintenance and growth. Bone density (levels of minerals) improves in response to load and you will strengthen bone all along the lines of stress through running. The inclusion of specific strength training exercises can also help by boosting bone density. It's worth knowing that bone remodels on a 6–12 month cycle so it may take time to notice the benefits.

TYPES OF STRENGTH TRAINING

Resistance training can be a concentric or eccentric contraction. Concentric exercise is a contraction that shortens a muscle as the joint angle is increased, while eccentric exercise is a contraction that lengthens the muscle as the joint angle is decreased. The eccentric part of the exercise is usually the return to the original position. An example is in a push-up, where the concentric element is the straightening of the arms as you push yourself up and the eccentric part is the lowering. Most exercises include both.

There are three key types of strength training:

1 ISOTONIC TRAINING This involves both concentric and eccentric movement, with the muscle changing in length. These are exercises designed to increase muscular strength, power and endurance through moving a constant amount of weight at variable speeds through a range of motion. These are typically pushing, pulling, lifting and lowering exercises, where the resistance is provided by gravity, weights or exercise equipment.

2 ISOMETRIC TRAINING These exercises involve neither concentric nor eccentric movement but employ a muscle that is held still. An obvious example of this is the plank, for which you remain in the push-up position for a period of time.

3 PLYOMETRIC TRAINING This usually involves different jumps, from the ground or from a height, provoking a rapid concentric movement of a specific muscle followed by a rapid eccentric movement. It helps produce a fast and strong muscle response. Often used to improve the flexibility and strength of particular muscle groups, but most of all to increase power.

MATCHING TRAINING TO DISTANCE

Building your own strength training programme will depend on your level of fitness in terms of training, which areas of your body are weakest and what your goals are in running. It will also vary according to which distance you are focusing on. *See* Chapter 15, pp. 215–219 for more information.

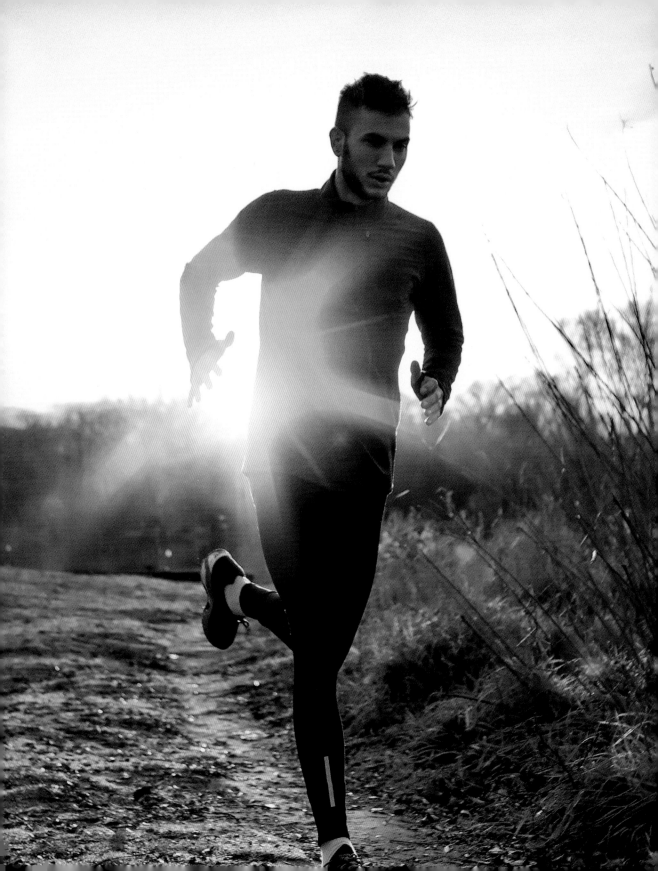

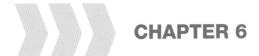

CHAPTER 6

ANATOMY AND PHYSIOLOGY

Anyone who has attended a physiotherapy session will know that the human body isn't a simple mechanism. Any explanation of problems in the Achilles, shins or knees is rarely confined to those areas. They are dependent on a structure of bones, joints and muscles which all have to play their part to avoid excess pressure being exerted at the weakest areas or points of stress.

The body contains 206 bones of all sizes, which give it shape and stability. Where each of the bones meet you will find a joint, which allows a degree of movement ranging from fixed to partially movable to free moving. The latter are cushioned by cartilage, which is a soft, spongy tissue, and connected by ligaments, which are a tough, fibrous and slightly elastic tissue that provides stability. Together, the bones and joints form a skeleton, the framework for muscles.

Although there are cardiac (heart) muscles and smooth (organ) muscles, it is the skeletal muscles that directly concern our movement. These are groups of fibrous tissues that are attached to bones by tendons and they are able to bunch up (contract) or relax to their normal size. In order to operate, muscles rely on other body parts, such as the brain, spinal cord and nerves, which transmit the signal to fibres in the muscle instructing them to contract. How powerfully they contract depends on the number of muscle fibres receiving the message.

When it does contract, the muscle gets shorter and pulls on the bone(s) it is attached to, making it abduct (move away from the body), adduct (move towards the body), rotate (pivot around a single axis) or circumduct (move in a circular pattern from a single point).

Muscle flexion and extension usually results in asymmetric movement. For example, when flexing the biceps, the lower arm (radius and ulna) move, but the upper bone (humerus) does not. Muscles can only pull or relax, they cannot push. Most muscles therefore work in pairs or groups (for example, the biceps flexes the elbow and the triceps extends it) and are aided by other muscles, which support the contraction or hold the rest of the body in place while the action happens. The effective operation of a muscle depends on several factors, some of which can be improved through training.

There must be an efficient neural pathway for the signals from the brain to the muscle through nerves, fibres and receptors. The adaptability of our nervous system is called 'neuroplasticity'. This is evident in how we adapt to learn a new skill such as back-heeling a football. As we repeat a new movement in a training programme (for example, one of the exercises contained in this book), our nervous system will improve its learning of the movement more quickly than the muscle will strengthen. Therefore, early signs of improvement will be down to the nervous system adapting, rather than the muscle strengthening.

The muscle must also be tough and strong. A runner's calves lift the heels about 1200 times every mile. Resistance exercises increase the diameter of muscle fibres, which builds muscle mass and strength and increases tissue elasticity. And, although aerobic exercise is the best way of improving muscles' efficiency in using oxygen and other energy sources, anaerobic exercise (like strength training) is effective for high-intensity activity such as sprinting.

Because opposing muscle groups work together to move the body they ideally need to be balanced. However, muscles in the front of the body (anterior) often become stronger than those in the back (posterior). For example, hamstrings are invariably weaker than quads, especially among those who have desk jobs or spend large periods of time seated. Runners often become 'quad dominant', overusing those muscles instead of the weaker hamstrings.

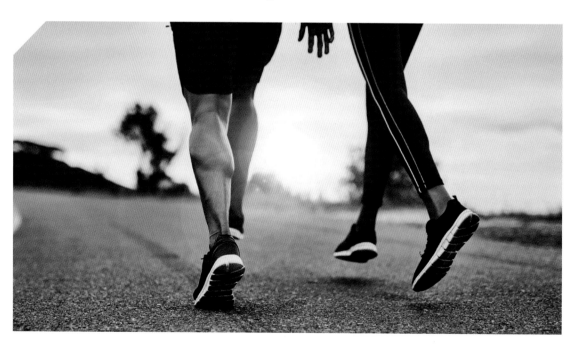

MAIN MUSCLE GROUPS USED IN RUNNING

The process of running involves an incredibly complex chain of co-ordinated muscle movement across the whole body and the activation of a number of large and small muscles in a specific sequence. Some are engaged in propelling the body forwards while others work to keep it upright.

In moving the leg forwards, the quadricep muscles at the front of your thigh are key. The largest and most powerful muscle group in the body, they help bend your hip and straighten your knee. The quads' opposing muscle group – the hamstring muscles that span the backs of the hips and thighs – are then employed in bending the knee and have a role in straightening the hip.

Quadriceps

Glutes

Hamstrings

As the foot hits the ground, the knee, calves, ankle and foot – supported by the quads and hamstrings – must all absorb the impact of landing. The calves and shins act as both brake and accelerator, controlling the landing and providing the spring power in pushing off. The forward propulsion includes the calf and also the mid-body, where the hip muscles and the famous 'glutes' – butt muscles – extend and then straighten the hip.

These muscle groups are therefore vital to running form and the ability to avoid injury and run faster. Each of the groups comprises completely different sets of muscles and an understanding of their function while running helps us to realise why looking after them is so important.

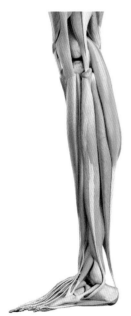

The key muscles of the lower leg

Calves

The calves are made up of three muscles — the medial and lateral gastrocnemius and the soleus — that run from just below the knee to the heel. The gastrocnemius is the most superficial (nearest the surface) of the calf muscles, with the soleus sitting deeper in the leg. They perform basically the same function, but the gastrocnemius attaches above the knee joint, while the soleus attaches just below. The distinction is important when stretching as the knee has to be straight when stretching the gastrocnemius and bent for the soleus. Not only is the soleus used more in everyday life – for example, for posture – but it is also often the calf muscle missed during stretching.

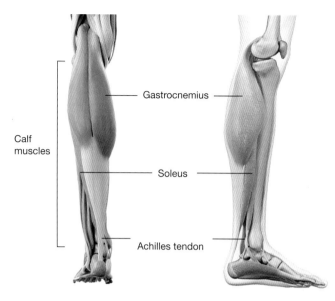

The basic job of these muscles is to raise the heel and point (plantarflex) the foot downwards. This is an extremely important component of the push-off and drive forwards. These are much smaller muscles than the quads, hamstrings and glutes, but they raise the heels around 1200 times every mile. Some studies have claimed the calves are required to work 25 per cent more than the quads. Unsurprisingly, they often become overworked and tired, which affects pace and stride and also means they provide less stability for the lower leg, putting additional stress on the Achilles, shins, hips and hamstrings.

The calf muscles have one more vital function: they are also the lower leg's circulation manager, sometimes grandly called 'the secondary heart', returning venous (used and deoxygenated) blood from the legs back to the heart. Each time the calf muscles contract, this forces about 70 per cent of the blood in the legs back towards the heart. When the calf muscles relax, the deeper veins in the legs are filled with blood.

Peroneus longus

If you feel the outside of your leg just below the knee, you will come across a small, lumpy bone: the head of the fibula. Try to follow the fibula down and it will disappear under a muscle: the peroneus longus. This muscle wraps round the ankle and its tendon attaches to the underside of the foot on the medial side. It is key to stabilising the foot and enabling it to become rigid for push-off. It is aided in this by the peroneus brevis muscle, which also originates on the fibula, but attaches to the base of the little toe. Together, the longus and brevis form half of a 'stirrup' around the foot. In conjunction with the tibialis posterior on the medial side, these muscles control and elicit inversion, eversion and plantar flexion in the ankle and foot.

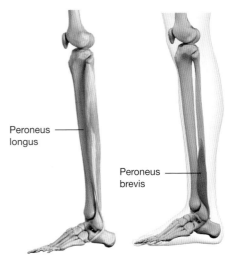

Peroneus longus

Peroneus brevis

When running, these muscles and tendons are put under stress in landing and in push-off. If the foot is hitting the ground on the outside of the foot (supination), they are forced to work on every step to maintain balance. They are also key in preventing the ankle from rolling inwards, but are often weaker than the muscles on the inside of the ankle. A loss of function here can lead to ankle sprains.

Tibialis anterior and tibialis posterior

The tibialis anterior runs down the front of the shin, just on the outside of the shin bone, with the tendon extending from the bottom of the shin diagonally across the ankle and attaching to the foot at the arch. Together with the tibialis posterior, it forms the second half of the foot stirrup with the peroneous muscles. Its main function is to dorsiflex the ankle — pulling your foot up towards your knee – but it also stiffens the ankle during mid-stance and creates inversion at the ankle joint that rolls the foot inwards.

The tibialis posterior muscle is embedded in the inner calf, but its long tendon runs down behind the ankle to the arch and anchors under the foot. As well as aiding the plantar flex and inverting the ankle, its main job is to help support the foot arch.

The tibialis anterior and the tibialis posterior are the muscles most associated with shin splints. When weak, the tibialis posterior is easily overloaded, particularly through overuse or when running downhill or on uneven surfaces. Weakness and injury can also be the result of poor muscle alignment or inadequate core stability.

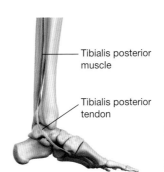

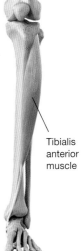

Tibialis posterior muscle

Tibialis posterior tendon

Tibialis anterior muscle

The gluteus muscles

The gluteus muscles, often called 'the glutes', are a muscle group located in each buttock. They are made up of three individual muscles – the gluteus maximus, the gluteus medius and the gluteus minimus – and play a major role in physical movement and stability. The gluteus maximus is the largest of these muscles and it is the primary muscle responsible for hip extension in running. The other glutes play their part by holding our pelvis level and steady and keeping the lower body aligned.

Medius

Maximus

Strong glutes are essential for athletes aiming to run faster. Not only is strong hip extension the basis of a powerful stride, but these muscles also restrict side-to-side movement, which produces a more efficient running style. Their strength is also fundamental to avoiding injury. Glute weakness is linked to Achilles tendinitis, runner's knee, iliotibial band syndrome (ITBS) and other injuries.

The major problem faced by many runners is that the glutes become inhibited – meaning they don't work to their full potential. This is generally because the gluteal muscles aren't as active as other muscles during daily life, and tight hip flexors resulting from hours spent sitting inhibit and weaken them. Then, when we run, we automatically look to stronger muscle groups – quads, hamstrings, calves – to contribute instead.

Hip flexors

The hip flexors are a group of seven muscles on each side of the body. They are found in the pelvic area and run from the the lower back via the hips and groin to the top of the femur (the long thigh bone, the strongest in the body). The main function of these muscles is to bring the knee towards the chest and bend the waist. Their strength and increased activity contribute significantly to an increase in speed as they drive the leg through the air to help lengthen the stride.

The principal hip flexors are the inner hip muscles that form the iliopsoas – a joint name for the merged iliacus and the psoas muscles. The psoas major is a deep-set, rope-like muscle that runs diagonally from the spine to the femur. At the hip, it merges with the iliacus, which extends to the thigh. The psoas works especially hard, contracting and lengthening at every stride, while the iliacus flexes and rotates the femur.

Great demand is placed on these muscles in particular, but despite being naturally strong they are often underdeveloped in many runners. So, often it is a stronger muscle that picks up the load. This can be the rectus femoris, one of the quadriceps, which crosses both the hip and knee joints, or the tensor fasciae latae, commonly referred to as TFL.

TFL is a small muscle found on the outside of the hip. It attaches at the top to the pelvis and runs down to connect to the iliotibial (IT) band, which acts as its tendon (albeit a very long, thick tendon). Its primary function is to rotate and stabilise the hip, but it is also called upon to support the small glutes and contribute to hip flexion. The versatility of such a small muscle presents problems; it can easily be overworked, but if inhibited, it can also put stress on other muscles, which rely on its support.

Sitting for long periods of time only serves to shorten and restrict the power the hip flexors are able to generate. Attention to developing all the hip flexor muscles is therefore key to improving both strength and performance.

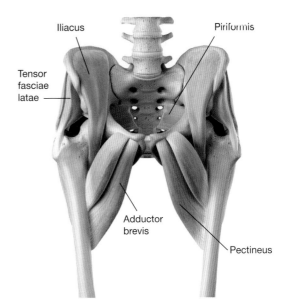

Iliacus

Piriformis

Tensor fasciae latae

Adductor brevis

Pectineus

The sartorius

The longest muscle of the body, the sartorius runs diagonally down the front of the leg, from the outside of the hip to the inside of the knee. Because it spans both the hip and the knee, it is involved in virtually every move you make with your lower body.

The sartorius is not the primary muscle in any action but it is important in providing support in hip flexion, hip adduction (taking a step sideways), external hip rotation (rotating the leg outwards) and knee flexion (bending the knee). A ribbon-like muscle, it is sometimes referred to as the 'tailor's muscle' – its name derives from the Latin word 'sartor' meaning tailor – perhaps related to the cross-legged position tailors once used to adopt.

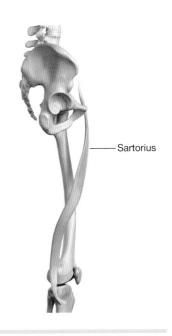

Sartorius

Pes anserinus

Just under the knee, at the tibia (shin bone), the sartorius joins two other muscles, gracilis and semitendinosus, at the pes anserinus. The gracilis is a muscle in the inside of the thigh used to pull the leg inwards, while the semitendinosus is a hamstring muscle used to pull your lower leg backwards and flex the knee. The tendons of these three muscles rub against a part of the tibia as the knee goes through its full range of motion so between the tendon and the bone is a lubricating sac called a bursa.

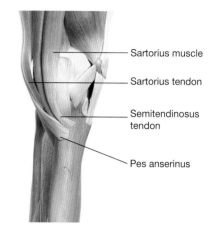

Sartorius muscle

Sartorius tendon

Semitendinosus tendon

Pes anserinus

The bursa is reasonably effective in reducing the friction on the tendons but, subjected to the continuous, repetitive actions of running, it can become swollen and tender and feel stiff or sore. The use of the sartorius can be seriously limited if this area gets inflamed, which of course impacts on other muscles throughout the lower body. Overuse is clearly the major factor in bursitis, but it can also be prevented by increasing the strength and flexibility of the surrounding muscles. Stretching exercises on the sartorius (*see* Hip Flexor Stretch, pp. 142–3), gracilis (*see* Hip Adduction, pp. 206–7) and semitendinosus will ensure they work smoothly with less friction.

The back

For all the work being done below the hips, it is so often the back that becomes the weak area for many runners. This is unsurprising when you consider the large and complex group of muscles that have to work together to support the spine, help hold the body upright and allow the trunk of the body to move and turn.

Much of the responsibility for the moving element of the job is assigned to the extensor muscles (attached to the back of the spine), the erector spinae (large paired muscles in the lower back) and the external obliques, part of the abdominals. Meanwhile, the essential task of keeping the body upright is down to the core muscles.

The deep core muscles include the pelvic floor muscles that help anchor the body at its centre; the transversus abdominis (TAs), a thick layer of muscle under the 'six-pack' area, which wraps around the torso from front to back and whose horizontal muscle fibres allow it to act like a corset or belt; the quadratus lumborum, a deep posterior abdominal muscle that runs from the pelvis up to the first rib and is essential in stabilising the pelvis; and the multifidus, a series of stabilising muscles attached to the length of the spinal column.

This neat arrangement breaks down when the muscles in and around the back are dysfunctional. Then the 'moving' muscles are forced to help stability and can overstretch and strain to compensate. This is especially true of tight hip flexors and weak back muscles – a common result of sitting for long periods of time. Tight hip flexors can pull the pelvis forwards (known as an anterior pelvic tilt), putting extra stress on the surrounding muscles, which results in lower back pain. The core will come under great pressure if the surrounding muscles are allowed to become light and weak. Or if the core is weak, the surrounding prime movers will have to do the job of the core as best they can. At some point they will overload and cause pain. Keeping a strong core and lower back muscles should be a key factor in your S&C programme.

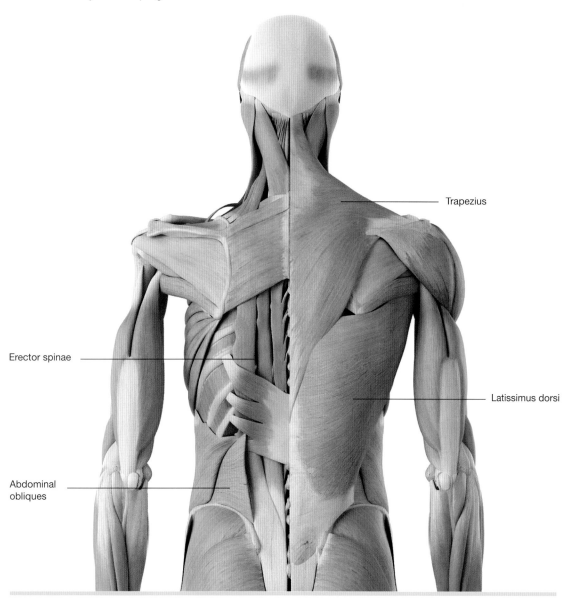

Trapezius

Erector spinae

Latissimus dorsi

Abdominal
obliques

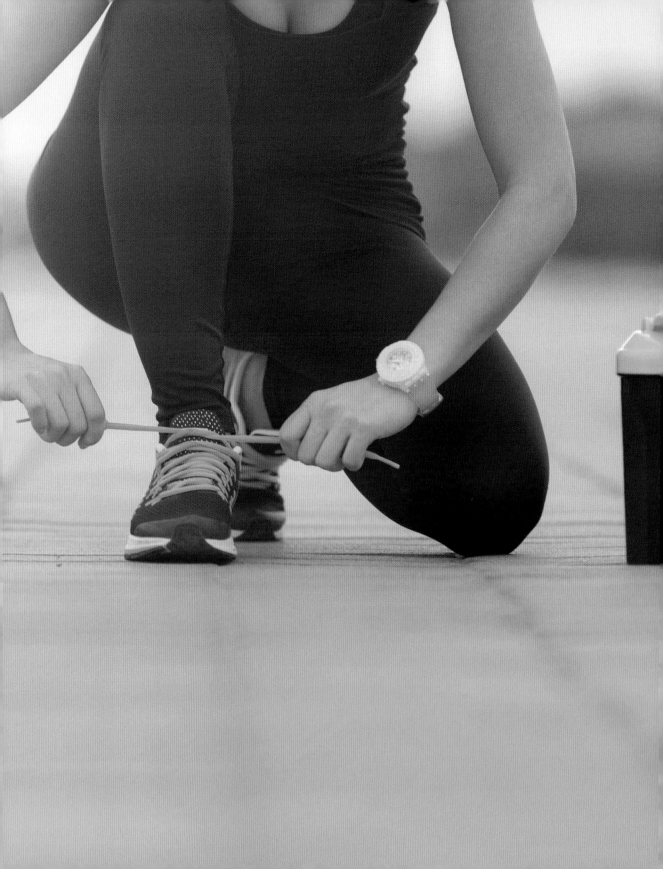

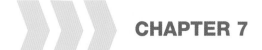
DIET AND NUTRITION

Physical activity and muscle growth is sustained by energy fuelled by what we consume, so diet is a hugely important consideration for any athlete. If we are to put our bodies under extra stress they need to have the carbohydrates, protein, vitamins, minerals and antioxidants to both undertake and recover effectively from any exercise. Although running, and indeed weight training, are often associated with specialised diets requiring manufactured supplements, the general rules of healthy eating and drinking require just minor adjustments to satisfy the extra physical demands.

HYDRATION

The average human body is 60 per cent water, so keeping a stable fluid balance in the body before, during and after physical activity is important, regardless of the nature of the exercise or the temperature. Our bodies require water to function, as it is an essential factor in circulation, regulating body temperature, the absorption of nutrients and supply of oxygen to cells, the digestive system and brain function.

Many of these functions directly affect us as runners and in our training. You will be familiar with the need to be fully hydrated when running, but it is essential for resistance training, too. The more fluid there is in your blood vessels, the easier it is for your heart to pump it to your cells and tissues. Also, studies have revealed that even mild dehydration (some researchers claim as little as 2.4 per cent) can cause the brain to send out messages to slow or stop.

Dehydration can adversely affect muscle endurance. Your body needs both water and electrolytes (sodium, potassium, magnesium, calcium and chloride) to support normal muscle contractions and if not replaced, the fluids lost through sweat can lead to tightening of muscles and an increased risk of strains and sprains. Cartilages consist of around 80 per cent water, which, along with synovial fluid, cushions the joints when they bear weight or pressure. Both of these also rely on full hydration for the recovery process as fluid levels and the blood circulation deliver the nutrients required to generate new cells.

How much water needs to be consumed depends on the individual, the temperature and the level of physical exertion.As I mentioned above, physical performance can begin to deteriorate at around 2.4 per cent dehydration levels, with the most rapid fall-off occurring at 5 per cent or greater. It is only at this point that you feel thirsty, so it is important to drink regularly –during as well as before and after exercise. The message here is when you feel thirsty, it's already too late, so drink little and often.

DIET

Given a healthy, balanced diet with plenty of vegetables and fruit and a reasonable intake of protein, fat and carbohydrates, our bodies can pretty much look after themselves. Any serious, or even semi-serious, runner should already have a sensible diet in which they consume the extra calories required to sustain their running schedule without putting on or losing weight. A strength training routine can be added to the schedule without a major rethink, although some considerations can be made that can aid muscle development.

Protein

Protein is necessary to build, maintain and repair muscle. Runners might already be consuming a substantial amount of protein in their diet but more might be needed to obtain the essential amino acids necessary for muscle synthesis after training and to minimise lean muscle being broken down for energy on training runs.

Runners embarking on a strength training programme should consider increasing their consumption to around 1.5g of protein per kilogram of body weight a day. For an average man weighing 65kg (145lb) that is around 100g (3½oz) of protein a day. Foods rich in protein include fish, chicken, tofu, eggs, beans and meat, but considering that there is approximately 50g (1¾oz) of protein in a chicken breast, 13g (½oz) in an egg and 20g (¾oz) in a cup of edamame beans, it is clear why including protein bars and drinks or whey powder can help supplement the diet.

Protein prolongs the period of increased insulin levels, which helps your body direct glycogen back into muscles and aids recovery. For this reason, it is advisable to consume some protein within 30 minutes of a workout. Palatable, portable and easy-to-digest, protein supplements are often seen as an ideal post-workout meal. Of course, creating low-sugar versions of these with naturally sourced ingredients may well be superior.

Vitamins and minerals

A diet containing fruits (especially berries and stone fruits) and a variety of vegetables will provide many antioxidant and anti-inflammatory vitamins and minerals that will help ease muscle soreness and limit injuries.

The following is a brief guide to how vitamins and minerals can help and where to find them:

❯ VITAMIN C Protects the body from exercise-induced oxidative stress, reducing muscle fatigue, inflammation and soreness.
Good sources include: green peppers, broccoli, blackcurrants and citrus fruits.

❯ VITAMIN D Helps the body absorb calcium, a vital component in muscle contraction.
Good sources include: oily fish, olive oil, cheese and eggs.

❯ VITAMIN K2 Plays a key role in bone metabolism and may help support bone health.
Good sources include: cheese, eggs, butter.

❯ VITAMIN B12 Helps ensure the brain and muscles communicate efficiently, which affects muscle growth and co-ordination.
Good sources include: meat, salmon, cod, milk, cheese, eggs.

❯ CALCIUM The calcium cycle enables contraction and relaxation of muscles. Lack of calcium can be the cause of cramps.
Good sources include: cheese, almonds, sesame seeds, sardines, yoghurt.

❯ POTASSIUM Has a role in transmitting electrical nerve impulses to signal muscle contractions.
Good sources include: bananas, oranges, grapefruit and dried fruits, such as prunes, raisins and dates.

❯ IRON Part of haemoglobin in blood and myoglobin in muscles, which help deliver oxygen to cells.
Good sources include: red meat, fish, grains, beans, nuts.

❯ MAGNESIUM Helps convert glycogen to glucose, thereby preventing accumulation of lactic acid and fatigued muscles.
Good sources include: spinach, dark chocolate, almonds, avocados.

❯ OMEGA 3 Improves muscle strength and function and reduces muscle damage and soreness.
Good sources include: mackerel, salmon, cod liver oil.

❯ NITRIC ACID Can increase blood flow and delivery of oxygen and nutrients to muscles.
Good sources include: beetroot, beet juice, watermelon, dark chocolate.

Supplements

Some runners are forever searching for that super-supplement that will transform their performance. Of course, it doesn't exist. Before reaching for any supplement, an athlete should look to their diet. The best nutrients come from a varied and healthy diet that includes a wide range of fruits and vegetables, whole grains, lean meats and dairy with natural, fresh and unprocessed food that retains nutrients and vitamins being a priority.

Recovery food is a good example. So many bars, shakes and other forms of supplement are promoted as the perfect recovery food following demanding training, but considering that an ideal recovery snack or meal simply needs to be rich in carbohydrates and include a source of protein, there is plenty of scope for homemade options. These might be Bircher muesli (oats soaked overnight in dairy with added fruit), a homemade smoothie (try adding tofu for added protein), a slice of toast with peanut butter and banana, or a homemade protein ball.

That said, there are some supplements that do warrant consideration. Athletes undertaking strength training routines should consider taking some form of multi-vitamin. Unless fruit and vegetables are truly organic, it is doubtful whether they contain sufficient vitamins and minerals. One report suggested that a single orange on sale in the 1950s may have held the same amount of vitamin A as 21 oranges bought from a supermarket today. It is therefore wise to take a daily soluble multivitamin pill, which will cover most of the essential nutrients listed above.

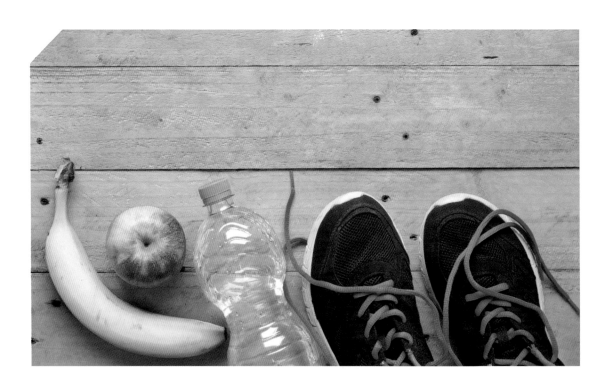

Diet and weight loss

Some run to lose weight faster and others lose weight to run faster. Both are possible and achievable but should be undertaken in moderation and with caution. Despite endless attempts to dress it up, the formula for weight loss is pretty simple: calories consumed need to be less than calories expended. Running isn't the most efficient way of burning calories, but it's not bad; a 10-km (6.2-mile) run can devour anything from 500 to 1000 calories.

However, your body needs to consume 2000–2500 calories to maintain weight. It can function normally with fewer calories, but at a certain point it will switch to survival mode, slowing down the metabolism and using body protein (from muscles) as fuel. This is not an ideal situation for a runner. The key to losing weight is to aim for a small reduction in calories – around 250 a day. You can do this by eating less, but alternatively, you could add five minutes to your strength training session (lean muscle burns about five calories per pound) or introduce interval sprints to a training run.

Calories are not the only concern for runners attempting to lose weight. The need to support training and recovery demands a different set of energy requirements to everyday living. Fad diets, which severely reduce consumption or exclude certain food groups, are particularly ill-advised. The rapid early weight loss that is a characteristic of many of them is largely body water. As explained earlier in this chapter, being sufficiently hydrated is an important part of the metabolism and dehydration can lead to electrolyte imbalance. Furthermore, runners undergoing strength training need a higher-than-average intake of carbohydrate, protein, vitamins and minerals. Deficiencies in any of these can lead to muscle breakdown.

Vegetarians, vegans and food intolerances

Whether it is for religious, ethical or health reasons, many runners will find their everyday diets can still fulfil the nutritional demands of running and training. It should be no barrier to undertaking a programme even up to elite level. Vegetarians will find it reasonably straightforward to modify portions and foodstuffs to ensure a suitably balanced diet. A protein shortfall is a possible problem, but beans, legumes, nuts, seeds and soy products are all viable alternatives as long as a wide variety of these are consumed to ensure a broad intake of different essential amino acids.

Vegan and lactose-intolerant athletes might find it more difficult, but the long list of high-achieving and world-class vegan runners proves it is not a major problem. It is just a matter of compensating for nutritional deficiencies. Calcium requirements may be matched with an abundance of green leafy vegetables and use of fortified dairy alternatives and tofu, nuts, seeds and grains can provide essential riboflavin (vitamin B2), though non-dairy consumers may wish to consider supplements for these.

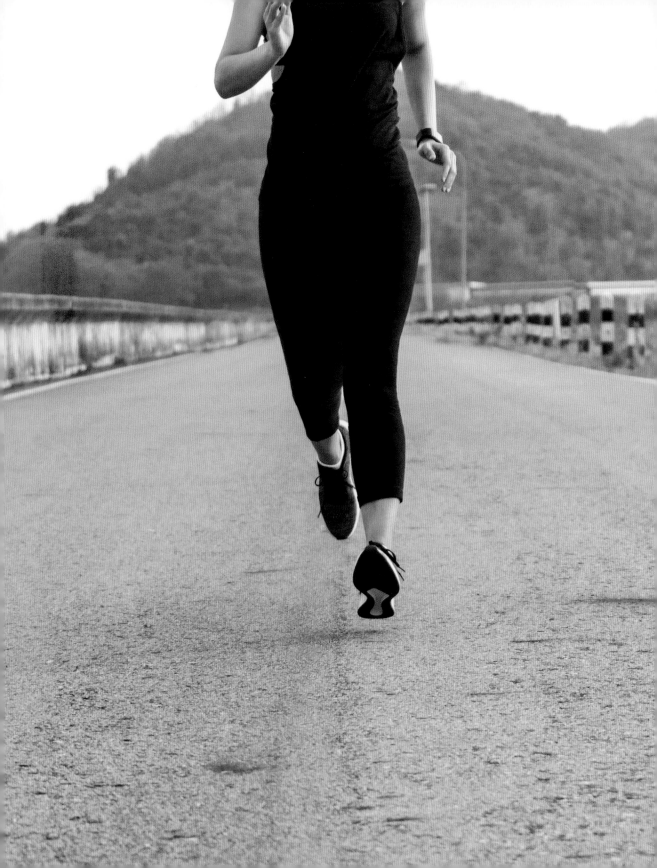

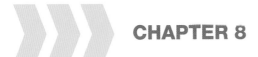

CHAPTER 8

BEFORE YOU START

Do you want to be a statistic? Most don't, unless it is to be the 'greatest' or 'best. But when it comes to looking after our bodies, only 7 per cent of runners actually do all the exercises prescribed by a physio. It's your choice: you can be part of the 93 per cent if you like and always participate in the negative statistics, or jump into the ever-growing 7 per cent group and change your horizons for the better.

So before you embark upon this lifestyle change and adopt a healthier outlook to preparation and injury prevention, consider that you will be a talisman for your running buddies. They will start to enquire as to how and why you are suddenly achieving better results, what training programme you are following or who is coaching you – they may even gossip that you are doping! Then with this great power comes great responsibility: do you tell them about this book and make me happy, knowing that you will level the playing field for your fellow runners, or do you keep it all a secret and enjoy the winning streak?

The choice is yours.

EQUIPMENT

The exercises in this book have been designed to be performed in your own home. If you have access to a gym and feel more comfortable working out there then fine, but all you really need is an uncluttered space with a flat, stable surface where you can move freely. All the stretches can be undertaken without equipment, but a small investment in kit will be necessary to perform the strength exercises. These items can all be purchased in sports outlets but may be less expensive through online retailers.

> **Exercise mat**
> A small outlay on an exercise mat is enough to prevent you having to lie on a cold, hard floor or leave sweat marks on your carpet. They provide a comfortable, non-slip and easy-to-wipe-down surface and will help focus your mind on your workout. Exercise mats tend to be thicker than yoga mats, but you don't need a super-dense version; a 1.5cm (0.6in) mat will suffice for the routines in this book.

〉 Towel

It's an item you might not have to purchase especially, but it is worth remembering to have a hand towel ready as part of your exercise equipment. It is used in some stretches to add basic resistance, as a stability tool or as a headrest.

〉 Resistance bands

Resistance bands are a relatively cheap (less than £20/$25 a set), but very effective piece of equipment. They are made of strong, thin rubber so as the band lengthens, the resistance increases. A set usually contains three or five different coloured bands with the colour of a band indicating the level of resistance. The middle range (usually red and green) bands will suit most people doing the exercises in this book. They are also available as tube bands with detachable handles, but the simple looped bands are sufficient for our purposes.

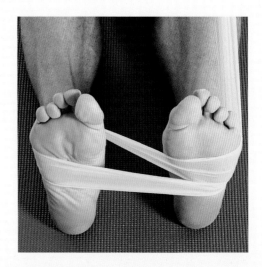

〉 Slant board

A slant board is a wedge-shaped construction often made of wood or foam and measuring around 30–40cm (12–16in) square and 15cm (6in) high. It provides an angled step; some are fixed at 20 degrees, others can be set at variable angles (either is fine for our purposes). It is used as an addition to a variety of stretching exercises as it is a great way of changing and increasing pressure on a host of different muscles and joints, especially the knees and calves.

〉 Dumbbells

Weights are an important feature of strength training. This doesn't mean the bar and hefty weights used by bodybuilders, but two lightweight sets (2kg/4.4lb and 4kg/8.8lb) of hand dumbbells. These are often used to add power to squats, twists and lunges.

〉 Marbles and bowl

This might seem an odd selection for exercise equipment, but toe exercises using marbles are a super-effective way of improving foot strength, especially in the plantar fascia and heel. All that is required is at least 20 small marbles and a bowl that's big enough to hold them.

❯ Swiss ball

Sometimes called an exercise ball, gym ball or even a stability ball, this is an inflated, soft elastic ball with a diameter of approximately 35–85cm (14–34in). It is a cheap but incredibly versatile training tool that enhances many routines. The key factor is its instability, which, of course, helps develop balance but also increases core strength and can develop muscles across the body.

Try to get one that is the right size for you. Here is a guide:

- 45cm (18in) ball for those who are 1.37–1.52m (4ft 5in–5ft) tall
- 55cm (22in) ball for those who are 1.52–1.65m (5ft–5ft 5in) tall
- 65cm (26in) ball for those who are 1.65–1.83m (5ft 5in–6ft) tall
- 75cm (30in) for everyone above that.

❯ Aerobic step

These are the plastic steps that are sold as 'aerobic steppers' as they feature heavily in aerobic workout routines. They are also ideal for strength training, particularly in calf raises. Though the basic versions available are perfectly adequate for the strength exercises here, it can be even better to find one with an adjustable height so that intensity levels may be increased.

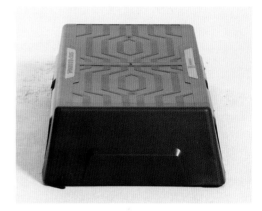

❯ Blood pressure cuff (optional)

Most modern blood pressure readers now come with a digital monitor and automatic inflator. However, much cheaper (around £10/$12) old-fashioned versions with a cuff, a ball to inflate and dial meter are still widely available. Sometimes referred to as an aneroid sphygmomanometer, this device can be used to measure core strength (*see* Chapter 9, pp.61–73), and aid the development of this important element of your training.

> " Only 7 per cent of runners do all the exercises prescribed by physios "

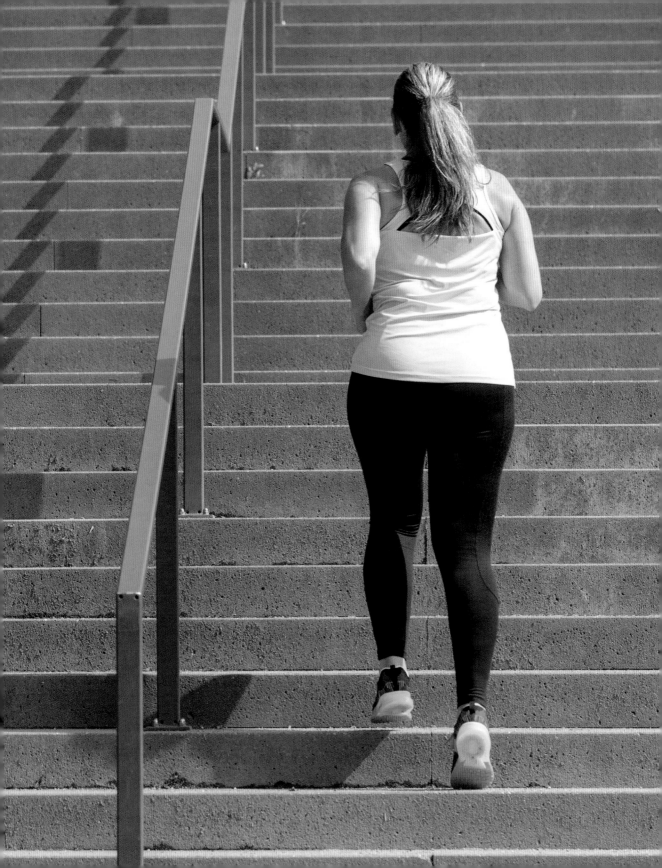

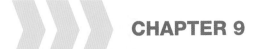

CHAPTER 9

CHECKING YOUR STRENGTH AND FLEXIBILITY

It is important to be able to assess what is needed for your own development and not to just blindly follow the stretches and strength training in this book. If you attempt to do this, then you will be spending most of your session doing exercises, some of which will be pointless and time-consuming, yielding no improvement in your performance or any reduction in your injury risk profile.

These tests are quite simple and repeatable. This section does not remove the need to see a specialist for a full assessment, but in the context of giving you some important information and a great start to your journey, it is vital that you do this if you want to get the most from this book. You *can* just read the book of course and spin past the bits you already know, but the devil is in the detail. I would wager that more than 90 per cent of you are working on your core incorrectly and have been for years, and that single-leg squats, if you're even doing them, are actually making your situation worse because of faulty technique. Remember, our aim here is for you to *do the basics well*. This book is not a complete brain dump of every advanced exercise I know! For best results, leave your ego at the door and do even the most straightforward exercise in an exceptional way.

HOW TO TEST AND MEASURE YOUR BODY

Start by doing each of these simple exercises. Look at yourself as you do them with a critical eye. Make sure you are taking the role of assessor and client at the same time, be open to criticism and trust the tests to find areas where you can improve rather than trying to confirm that you are already the finished article. I only say this as I have worked with so many runners and have learned that running ability is a poor correlation for good technique or strong biomechanics.

For instance, I have come across total beginners who are run-walking on a couch-to-5km course for the first time who have superior core strength to those who can run 5km in under 20 minutes. I have seen Olympic runners unable to perform a knee-to-wall test for their ankle flexibility and yes, they had numerous injuries in the area. So you see the purpose of the test is to establish what needs to be worked on and then we can put your efforts in the right place and make best use of time.

Think of yourself as a buckled bicycle wheel, where some of the spokes are too tight and some too loose. The engineer needs to tighten (strengthen) some and loosen (stretch) others for the wheel to obtain balance and optimal function again. So let's find out by testing which of your spokes is causing the issues and then let's concentrate on just those areas. This means you may have to resist the temptation to stretch both hamstrings for a while and just work on one side. As crazy as that will seem to you, it's important to get everything equal first before working on developing your body for optimal performance.

Calf muscles: soleus

1 Stand facing a wall and rest your hands on the wall at shoulder height.
2 Place one foot so the toes are close to the wall (skirting board) and check that your knee can touch the wall without your heel lifting off.
3 Keep sliding your foot backwards away from the wall and checking if the knee can still touch the wall with the heel down. You have reached your maximum when your toes are as far away from the wall as possible and you can touch the knee to the wall without lifting your heel from the floor at all.
4 Measure the distance between your toes and the wall and compare left to right. Record the distance using the table below.

DATE	LEFT	RIGHT

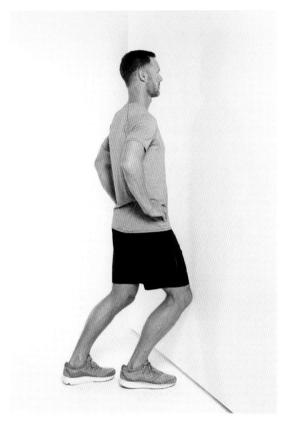

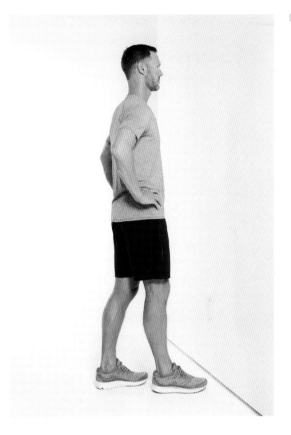

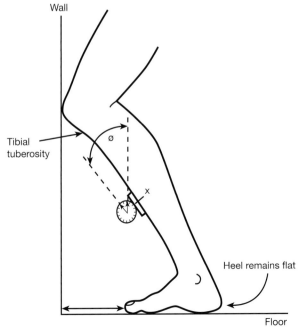

Wall

Tibial tuberosity

ø

x

Heel remains flat

Floor

Single-leg squat (SLS)

1 The test for a single-leg squat is simple, but difficult to measure accurately. The best way is to do it in front of a full-length mirror. Run a strip of masking tape down one side of the mirror to create a ruler. Use this to measure or mark the depth of your hips on your SLS.

2 Stand a repeatable distance away from the mirror (so you can test 'self against self' with some accuracy) and then, facing the mirror, perform a single-leg squat.

3 The single-leg squat is an art form; it's easy to cheat and lose sight of what you are trying to do. Hips must remain level and the knee needs to sit in a fine line of two axis points. It must not deviate medially or laterally, but remain over the middle toe, while also not extending beyond the end of your foot. The height you can dip down with all three of these parameters in check is the height of your single-leg squat. Choosing to dip lower just compounds faulty technique and will impact your running. As soon as the knee starts to deviate towards the midline, stop. Take a guess as to which line your knee reached on your masking tape scale.

4 Now place a horizontal line of tape at this point, then go back to your mark and retest. It will now be easier to tell if you have the correct height as you will see if your knee reaches the same point. Take your time to get this measurement

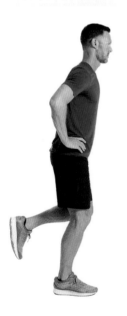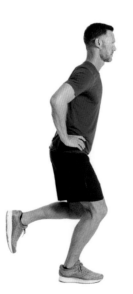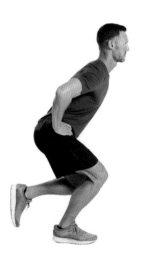

accurate for left and for right, but do not obsess (yes, I know runners well!) over it. Leave the tape on the left-hand side of your mirror with the height of your left knee depth and do the same for the right. You will use these daily for your exercises, but you'll also need to move them weekly as you progress, so be prepared to leave your set-up there indefinitely, without anyone in your house moving anything.

It is quite normal to find people cannot dip lower than 5cm (2in) at first, so work to a level that is easy for you to achieve and don't try to be a hero with this exercise. Starting at an easier level will allow you faster progression in a few weeks.

DATE	LEFT	RIGHT

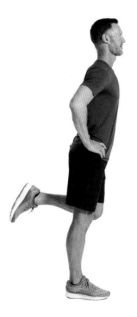
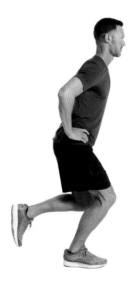

Bridge with single-leg lift

The bridge is a core, balance and glute exercise all rolled into one. It's a great test of these three parameters, but core especially. Core is not your six-pack by the way (however well hidden that might be) – it is the natural corset that surrounds the whole of the lower spine, including the transverse abdominus, thoracolumbar fascia, multifidus, internal and external obliques, rectus abdominus, erector spinae and diaphragm.

So, when doing this test, it is measuring the coactivation of all of these muscles and the glutes, hamstrings, etc as well.

1 Lie on your back on a firm surface, perhaps on an exercise mat, with your knees bent and feet flat on the floor (think old-fashioned sit-up start position). Put your arms out to the side like a crucifix.

2 Now slowly lift your hips up so that you have alignment through from the shoulders to the knees.

3 Maintain the straight line from shoulder to knee and extend one leg so the thighs are still in line, but now one leg is straight. You need to keep the straight line through your body, hips in line and no twist from left to right. Now do the same with the other leg. As with all these tests, you need to be strict. It might be worth enlisting the help of a friend or family member who can look to see if you are maintaining the alignment or not. If your core is losing control, you will start to feel the hamstrings cramping or overworking, or the lower back will start to ache and overtense.

You should be able to hold this position without any adverse effects for 30 seconds. If you can't then you need to go back to working the deep core, refer to transverse abdominus activation with blood pressure cuff (*see* p. 68) and glute activation (*see* p. 70) before returning to this test.

4 **INTERMEDIATE** If you are successful, try the intermediate level exercise: bring your arms into your sides and repeat. If you cannot maintain equilibrium of all angles here then work the basics as above plus the bridge with arms out until you can.

5 **ADVANCED** The advanced level, which everyone should be aiming for, is to be able to do this test with your arms folded over your chest.

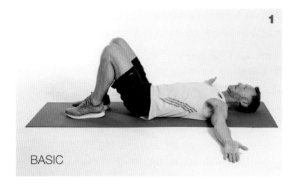

BASIC

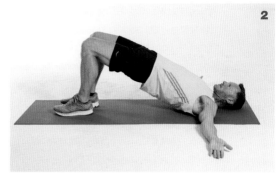

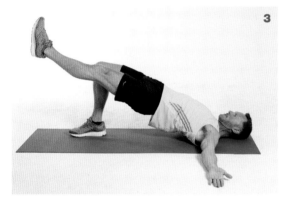

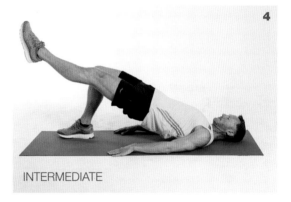

INTERMEDIATE

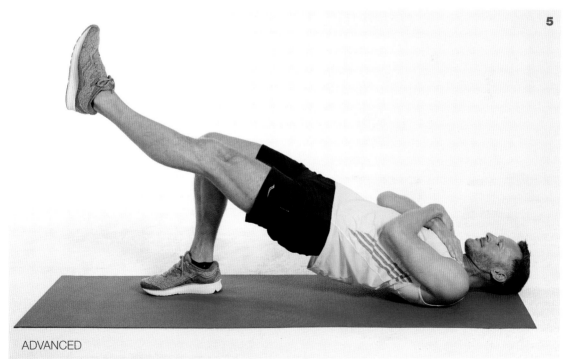

ADVANCED

Transverse abdominus activation with blood pressure cuff

The transverse abdominus muscles are the key core muscles you need to assess here. When strong, they offer a great deal of support to the lumbar spine. This is because when you activate the transverse abdominus muscles, you are in turn coactivating the natural corset of muscles that wraps around your body – transverse abdominus, thoracolumbar fascia, multifidus, internal and external obliques, rectus abdominus, erector spinae and diaphragm.

This test requires some equipment, notably an aneroid sphygmomanometer blood pressure cuff (*see* p. 59).

1   Lie on your back on a firm surface, perhaps on an exercise mat, in the crook lying position (like an old-fashioned sit-up, with bent knees and feet flat on the floor).

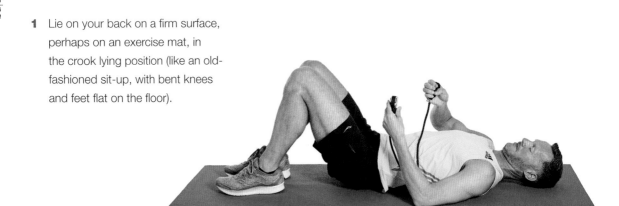

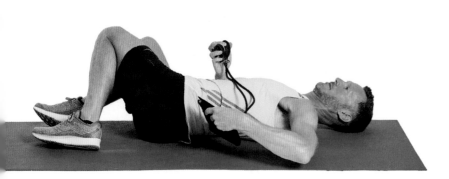

2   Place the deflated blood pressure cuff under the small hollow in your lower back, lock the air vent and press the little hand pump until it inflates to a millimetre mercury level of 40mmHG. Let the cuff settle for a few seconds; you may need to adjust it a few times until it is on 40mmHG (especially if it is brand new).

3 Now you need to activate your core. You do this by following these three simple steps.

    I. Imagine you are going to the toilet and you stop the flow. You will feel the muscles in your lower abdomen on each side tense and the mmHG will rise a bit.

    II. Draw in your belly button towards the spine by using the abdominal muscles and not through breath holding. You can check by holding this for a minute and seeing if you need to breathe suddenly, or simply try talking through the process.

    III. Gently press your lower back into the blood pressure cuff.

With all three of these activation steps in place you will notice the mmHG will have risen. It is your job to hold the needle at 70mmHG.

You may find that the needle is too high or too low. Try going through each of the steps until you have a coactivation of all the core muscles and the needle is steady on 70mmHG.

4 Now comes the test. You need to maintain the 70mmHG and lift one foot slowly off the floor, maintain the same 70mmHG and then lower the foot back down again. As soon as one foot touches back down the other must lift off.

You need to be able to repeat the process 25 times without the needle jumping all over the place.

It takes most people weeks to achieve this though, so see it as a process of hard work for the next few weeks. It is not for the faint-hearted and requires dedication. The weakest points are at the change of direction when the foot leaves the floor, the end of the leg lift and the change of direction when the foot returns to the floor. Pay close attention at these points and watch for a needle moving.

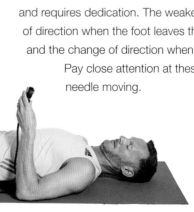

Glute activation

The glute muscle needs to be activated at the same time as the hamstring or just before. It is the prime hip extensor but becomes underutilised and overstretched from too much sitting and the resultant overactivity and tightening of the hip flexors. This is known as glute amnesia. If your glutes have it, we need to wake them up again.

1 To test, you need a helpful assistant. Lie on your front, ideally on a flat surface that is slightly raised so that you can drop your feet off the end; this can't be a bed as it will likely be too soft.

2 Ask your helpful assistant to place three fingertips on your glute and four on your hamstring and gently press down so they can feel the muscle.

3 Now lift your leg straight up (important: no knee bend) and your assistant can tell you if your glutes or hamstrings fired first. By firing, we mean which pushed on their fingers first. The temptation for you to tense your glute to prove you are doing this right will be high, but that ruins the test. Remember, you want to learn what's working, not try to prove a point.

4 After one leg lift, relax all your muscles, then repeat again up to five times. Your assistant will be able to monitor if the result is the same or changes over time.

5 Use the table below to record your results.

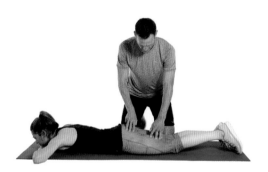 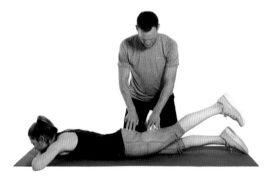

GLUTE ACTIVATION RECORD										
ACTION	LEFT-SIDE TESTS					RIGHT-SIDE TESTS				
	1	2	3	4	5	1	2	3	4	5
Glute before hamstring										
Hamstring before glute										
Together										

Hamstring length

1 Using a helpful assistant again, lie on your back, ideally on a flat surface that is slightly raised.

2 Ask your assistant to lift one leg up, with a bent knee, until the thigh is at a comfortable angle to the torso.

3 Keeping the thigh in this position, ask them to slowly start to straighten the leg by pushing up the foot towards your head.

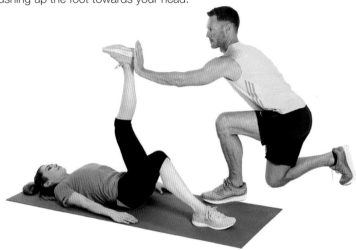

When the tension is such that the leg cannot easily be pushed any further (make sure they know to stop and not force the leg), they should take a measurement of the angle. Physiotherapists are accustomed to doing this using sight alone and science has shown this to be incredibly accurate compared to someone using a goniometer (angle measure ruler). I therefore suggest that your assistant judges the angle by eye, imagining a straight leg to be 180 degrees and working backwards from there. If you want to be in a more accurate test-retest situation at home then there are free apps available for your smartphone that do the job perfectly. There's a new device called the EasyAngle® that has made this process very easy for healthcare professionals.

HAMSTRING LENGTH RECORD		
	LEFT	**RIGHT**
Knee angle		

Overhead squat

1 Take a towel or broom handle and hold it in both hands above your head with straight arms in a Y position.
2 Perform a squat down to a level where the thighs go beyond parallel to the floor.

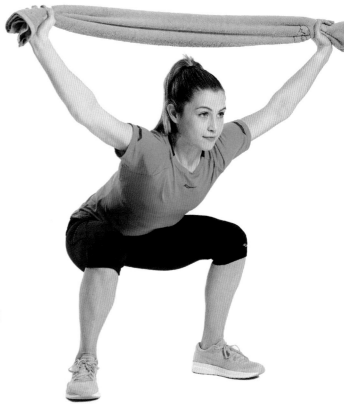

You need to be able to keep your hands above your head, maintain balance and and keep your heels on the ground.

An inability to do all of these things shows a weakness and imbalance in the links between the upper and lower body, a lack of ankle and hip mobility, and issues through the whole back. Notice what is tight or painful and work on those muscles from the exercises in this book. After six weeks of practice, retest.

Upper body wall slides

The upper body wall slide is an effective measure of the upper body in relation to the overhead squat you have just performed. This test will help differentiate between the upper and lower body limitations revealed by the overhead squat test.

1 Stand with your head, upper back and glutes against a wall. Place both of your hands and arms against the wall, elbows bent to 90 degrees and forearms going straight up (think of a pea on a fork).
2 Keep your lower back and legs against the wall and do not allow yourself excessive curves in your back as you slide your elbows down towards your sides as far as you can.
3 Now, raise your arms up as high as they will go. Concentrate on keeping your arms, elbows and shoulders against the wall as well as your back and legs.

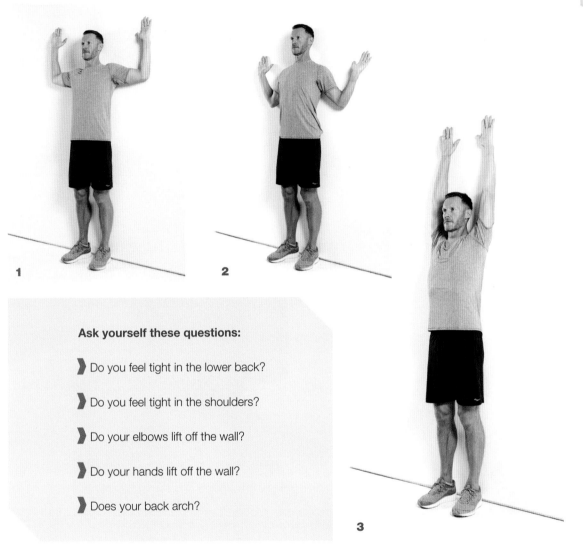

1

2

3

Ask yourself these questions:

❯ Do you feel tight in the lower back?

❯ Do you feel tight in the shoulders?

❯ Do your elbows lift off the wall?

❯ Do your hands lift off the wall?

❯ Does your back arch?

Write down all the things that happen and how you feel. If the answer to more than two of the statements above is 'yes' then consider doing some upper body mobility exercises. This will assist your running in many ways: better technique, improved posture, breathing will become easier and you will run faster. The following exercises will be of use: IJWTYH (*see* pp. 130–1) and Thread the Needle (*see* pp. 122–3) plus the internal and external rotation of your shoulder in Arm Circles (*see* pp. 126–7).

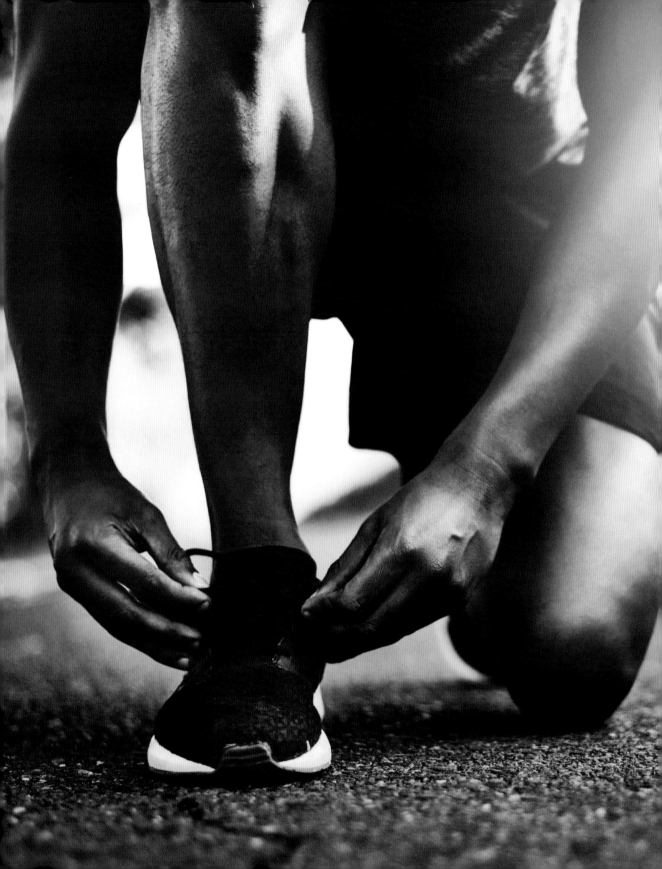

CHAPTER 10

REDUCING INJURY

It's no secret that running can take its toll on a body. Some studies claim as many as 75 per cent of runners suffer some kind of injury over a year. Accidents, ill-fitting footwear and congenital deficiencies account for some, but most are caused by overuse; a heavy training schedule, long-distance running or large increases in training intensity can all put repetitive stress on joints and muscles.

An overstretching of fibres in the muscle or the tendon is at the heart of most overuse injuries. When these fibres are subjected to stress, they sustain small micro-tears. The body can usually manage these and quickly repair the damage. However, in cases of sudden or repetitive stress, the rate or extent of the repair exceeds the body's immediate healing capability. The simple argument for strength training is that the stronger the muscle fibres, the more stress they can endure and the less likely they are to strain or tear.

Although by no means comprehensive, the following describes the most common injuries sustained by runners and how a strengthening of key muscle groups is often the best means of preventing injury. A more in-depth look at this information can be found in my previous book, *Running Free of Injuries*.

PLANTAR FASCIITIS

The plantar fascia is a flat length of connective tissue that runs from your heel bone (calcaneus) to the base of your toes (it splits into five 'digital slips', one for each toe). Its main roles are supporting the long arch in the foot and helping with the 'toe off' (see p. 15). Plantar fasciitis is an injury to this band of tissue, a stubborn condition often characterised by pain in the base of the heel or along the arch of the foot (usually, but not always, just on one foot).

Plantar fasciitis is often felt in the first few steps of the morning or after you've been sitting down for a while. It can be painful at first but becomes more of a dull ache once you have warmed up. Preventative training focuses on the weak and tight muscles and tendons that should support the foot.

ACHILLES TENDINOPATHY

The Achilles tendon, which connects the calf muscles to the back of the heel, is the thickest and strongest tendon in the body. Tendinopathy is a broad definition taking in a number of conditions that can cause pain in this area.

Sufferers feel stiffness in the back of the lower leg or above the heel, often first thing in the morning. Symptoms usually improve with light activity, but during a run, a mild ache can develop into more severe pain with prolonged training. The key to preventing injury to this area is the calf raise. Strengthening calf muscles and using a graded loading programme really helps avoid injury to this area.

SHIN SPLINTS

The bane of many runners, shin splints – or medial tibial stress syndrome (MTSS) – is a sharp pain just off the inside edge of the lower tibia by the calf muscles. The pain is caused by repetitive impact and strain on the shin and surrounding tissues, especially the two tibialis muscles, which leads to inflammation in the periosteum – the fibrous outer layer of the bone. The pain can be concentrated in a small 5cm (2in) area or spread further along the length of the shin bone.

Shin splints are more prevalent in novice or less fit runners as muscles do not develop in size, strength and flexibility at a sufficient rate to bear the load of regular

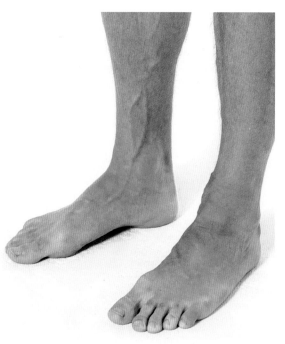

running. Exercises can strengthen the tibialis muscles themselves, but just as important are the calves, abductors and hip muscles, which all help stabilise the tibia on each impact.

ANKLE SPRAINS

The versatility and flexibility of the ankle has its drawbacks: the foot can easily roll unnaturally, overstretching or even tearing the ligaments of the ankle. Most sprains are lateral (accounting for 25 per cent of all running injuries), whereby the foot rolls outwards, affecting the three small ligaments on the outside of the ankle.

The consequences of ankle sprains are familiar to most runners: a swollen and bruised area that can be localised to a golf ball-sized swelling on the outside ankle bone, or a swollen area the size of a trainer sock, depending on the severity. This will be accompanied by throbbing or searing pain even when the ankle is not bearing weight. Often the cause is unavoidable – an unseen hole or bump in the terrain – but an unbalanced running gait can also be a contributory factor, as can a weakness of control of the gait cycle.

Most useful for prevention are exercises that are specifically designed to strengthen those muscles surrounding the ankle – the calves, the peroneal muscles that run down the outside of the lower leg and the tibialis posterior (shin) – as well as routines that improve balance or proprioception (the sense of knowing where a body part is in space at any particular time).

METATARSAL STRESS INJURIES

The metatarsal bones – five long, thin bones in middle of the foot that connect the ankle to the toes and give the foot its arch – are particularly vulnerable to repetitive pressure. Unfortunately, they take much of the impact on foot strike and can easily become strained, inflamed or fractured. Stress reaction in the bone is first evident by an increasing pain on movement, which abates when at rest. It is marked by tenderness to the touch and swelling on the top of the foot over the bones.

Another overload injury, a metatarsal stress fracture is usually caused by increasing running distance, frequency or speed too quickly. Reasons for the injury might include foot posture, badly-fitting footwear and poor running technique, but often it comes down to a significant increase in training, or lack of strength and flexibility in the hips, legs, ankles and feet. Strengthening glutes, quadriceps, calves and core stabilisers will all aid prevention, while as bones strengthen in relation to their surrounding muscles, working on toe flexors, plantars and peroneous muscles will help to fortify the metatarsals.

MORTON'S NEUROMA

This sometimes painful condition affects the ball of the foot. It can feel as if your socks are bunching up or even that you have a small stone in your shoe, and it may be accompanied by a sensation of pins and needles in the toes. A neuroma is a thickening of the tissue that surrounds the nerve leading to the toes and most frequently develops between the third and fourth toes. It affects women almost 10 times more often than men and can be caused by overload, overpronation and other biomechanical asymmetries, or even by wearing tight-fitting shoes.

Reducing pressure on the arch of the foot is fundamental to avoiding Morton's neuroma. This includes stretches to the lower leg, especially the calf and Achilles muscles, and strengthening the plantar fascia and other foot muscles can also decrease the stress in that area. However, footwear that allows the toes to spread out may offer a lot of relief.

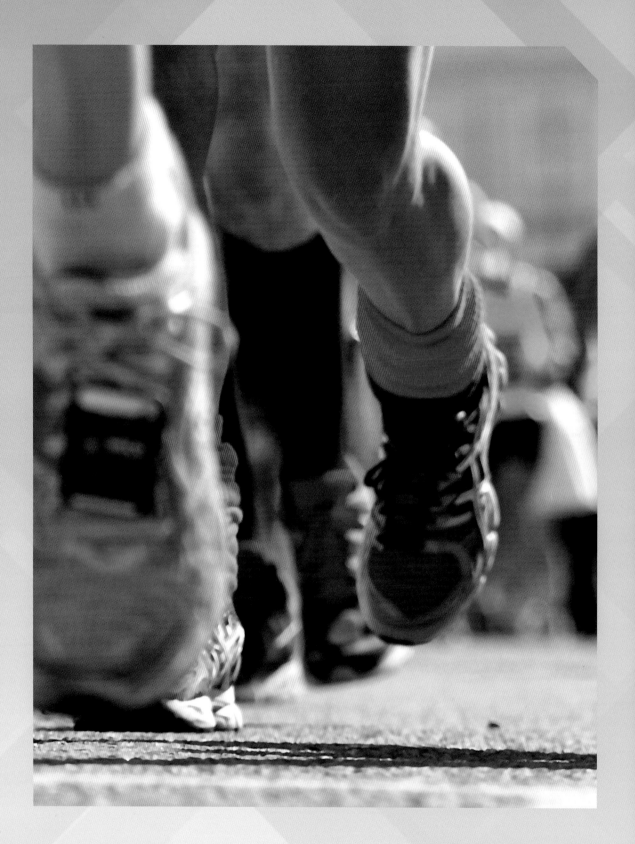

CALF STRAIN OR TEAR

A calf strain involves damage to one or more of the muscles in the lower leg (gastrocnemius, soleus or plantaris). It can affect fibres within the muscle or where the muscle joins the Achilles tendon. The calf performs a fast and large contraction when running. As the foot pushes off the ground, the calf can stretch beyond its ability to withstand the tension, and the resulting stress on the muscle may result in a strain or, if extreme, a tear.

Damage to the muscle tissue can result in inflammation, causing pain, soreness and tightness along the back of the lower leg. It can be felt as a dull ache experienced when running or a sharp pain even when walking, depending on the severity of the injury. Obviously, any strengthening of the calf muscles will help them bear a greater load, but the glutes also contribute to push-off and if strengthened, they can relieve the calves of excess stress.

RUNNER'S KNEE

Runner's knee is the common term used to describe pain around or under the patella (kneecap). The pain and stiffness it causes when bending the knee can make it difficult to climb stairs or even walk. Known medically as patellofemoral pain syndrome, it is caused by the patella failing to run smoothly in the trochlear groove – a small channel at the end of the femur. Factors causing this include overuse, overpronation and a malpositioned patella, but recent research has highlighted how far the knee travels inwards mid-stance (when the body is over the foot) as a major issue – women suffer more as their knees move more medially.

Injury might well be prevented by strengthening the knee's surrounding muscles. The quadriceps play a major role in controlling of the knee, while the hip muscles maintain a level pelvis. If weak, they allow the pelvis to drop on the opposite side as you bend the knee, placing extra stress on the knee's tracking.

ITBS

The ITB – iliotibial band – is a thick, fibrous band of tissue that runs laterally down the length of the thigh, from the gluteus maximus and tensor fasciae latae (TFL) to the tibia, just below the knee. It works with the knee ligaments to keep the knee aligned and to control unwanted movement. ITBS ('S' for 'syndrome') occurs when the ITB is overworked as it attempts to maintain the alignment. The glutes and the TFL tighten, pulling the ITB tight against the knee joint and causing it to rub repeatedly. This friction causes a stabbing sensation or ache on the outside of the knee, which can spread further up or down the leg or even to the hip. The pain will cease when running stops, but increases with further movement.

As the ITB is connected to the glutes, any weakness in these muscles can contribute to decreased stability in the knee, allowing it to be pulled too far inwards or outwards. Modern sedentary living leaves many people with underdeveloped glutes and thus more prone to ITBS, so strengthening these muscles, along with the hips, is an effective preventive action.

PATELLAR TENDINOPATHY

The patella tendon is a short but very wide tendon that runs from the patella to the top of the tibia (shin). It works with the muscles at the front of the thigh to extend the knee when running. A problem with this tendon can result in a mild stiffness of the knee or a sharp pain below the kneecap, felt especially when running downhill or descending stairs (unlike runner's knee, it does not hurt along the top or the side of the kneecap).

Patellar tendinopathy is usually an overuse injury, caused by repeated stress on the tendon. Prevention centres around working the quads and hamstrings, which will decrease strain on the tendon, strengthening thigh muscles that help control descents and ensuring a muscular balance to check the pull of stronger muscles on the tendon.

PES ANSERINE BURSITIS

The pes anserinus (see p. 48) is an attachment point of three muscles (sartorius, gracilis and semitendinosus) and is found on the inside of the knee joint, just behind the shin. It is the source of pain for runners as a result of a change to either the tendons themselves, or a bursa (small sack of fluid), which cushions the tendons and the bone. Both tendinopathy and bursitis in the area are characterised by a spontaneous then gradually worsening pain in the inner knee, below the kneecap level.

With three active muscles being responsible for the inward rotation and bending of the knee joint, it is a vulnerable area. Friction between tendons, bursa and bone is often a result of overwork due to weak muscles in the knees, upper legs and abdomen. Therefore, strengthening the adductors, quads and hamstrings is key to preventing injury in this area.

> **"The stronger the muscle fibres, the more stress they can endure and the less likely they are to strain or tear"**

QUADRICEPS TENSION

The four quadriceps muscles are located at the front of the thigh. They are essentially knee extensors – the muscles that straighten the bent knee. Aside from occasional 'morning after' discomfort in the thighs after a long run, runners do not suffer much pain in the area. However, tight quadriceps can pull on the kneecap, forcing it out of true alignment. They can also affect the hamstrings, hip joint and hip flexor muscles, causing pain and discomfort when walking, and cause the pelvis to tip and pull down, resulting in lower back pain and postural problems.

Those who are overly active or too sedentary are most vulnerable to tight quads. Overtraining is a key factor, but sitting at a desk all day creates muscle tension in the quads as they are in a nearly contracted position. Regular stretching and strengthening using lunges, squats and so on is an obvious prevention technique, but so is building strength in the glutes and other surrounding muscles as that puts less pressure on the quads to overcompensate for weak muscles.

HIP FLEXOR ISSUES

The hip flexors are a group of muscles that are active throughout the running cycle, driving the leg up and forwards in the swing phase and controlling motion during the push-off. Tight hip flexors can be caused by overuse, but once again extensive sitting is a more likely cause. In a sitting position, the hip flexors shorten, but still work to maintain posture. If they become overused or overstretched during running, the psoas muscle's tendon or the iliopsoas bursa can become inflamed, resulting in a painful swelling.

Immobility of the hips can be a major contributor to pain in other parts of the body. If the hip lacks the mobility to turn inwards as the foot turns, considerable stress is put on the knee. Tight hip flexors also cause an unnatural curve of the spine called hyperlordosis, which results in pain and soreness in the lower back. To counter any weakness, hip flexors can be targeted with specific stretches, but strengthening the glutes, abdominal muscles and hamstrings will ensure less pressure is being put on this area.

HIGH HAMSTRING TENDINOPATHY (HHT)

This common and debilitating condition is pretty unique to runners as it focuses on the hamstrings at the back of the thigh – an often weak group of muscles that are nevertheless integral in the running cycle. The critical area is where the tendons of the hamstring muscles attach to the sit bone (ischial tuberosity) at the base of the pelvis in the buttock. Adverse load at this site causes tendinopathy and can also irritate the bursa.

High hamstring tendinopathy develops slowly, but can become a nagging and chronic pain in one or both buttocks. Strength training of the hamstrings is an obvious guard against HHT, but working on the hip muscles – glutes and the lateral rotators – will lessen the dominance of the hamstrings when running and reduce hip adduction and internal rotation, contributors to the heavy load on the sit bone.

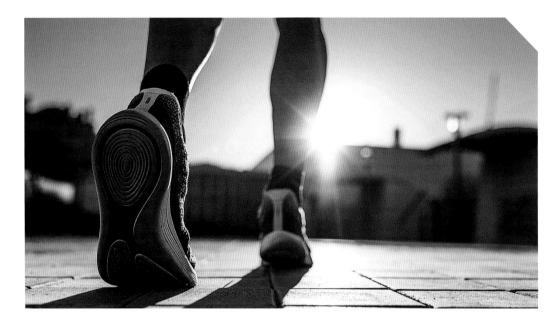

HAMSTRING STRAINS AND TEARS

As well as their tendons, the hamstring muscles are an area of potential injury for runners. The tendons or muscles can be stretched beyond their limit as a result of explosive movements such as sprinting or lunging, but more often because of gradual and repeated overstretching. Pain and tenderness is felt at the back of the thigh and it can become painful to move the leg.

As with HTT, prevention of hamstring injuries is helped by increasing intermuscular co-ordination (all the fibres in the muscle contracting and relaxing in sync) of the hamstring muscles themselves, strengthening of the glutes to contribute effectively in the running cycle and enabling the hip muscles to exert pelvic control.

GLUTEAL TENDINOPATHY

While glutes have been shown to be a key muscle group in various injuries, they can also be a source of pain in themselves. The gluteal tendons are the tough fibres that connect your gluteal muscle to your hip bone. As these muscles enable the hip to abduct and stabilise the pelvis, the glute tendons can easily be overstressed, especially among runners with poor hip and gluteal muscle control.

Injuries are usually cumulative, but hip pain can come on quite suddenly, along with muscle stiffness and a loss of strength in the hip muscles. Pelvic stability and reduced load on the hip is again key to avoiding injury and is achieved through exercises that strengthen the glutes and other hip muscles.

PIRIFORMIS SYNDROME

The piriformis is a band-like muscle located in the buttock, running from the sacrum at the base of the spine to the top of the femur (thigh bone). It helps stabilise the hip joint and lifts and rotates the thigh away from the body. If overworked, it tightens, putting pressure on the sciatic nerve, which it overlies. Often mistakenly self-diagnosed as sciatica, piriformis syndrome shares its symptoms of referred pain along the backs of the legs, in the buttocks or even in the lower leg and feet.

Heavy and consistent mileage by runners is a common cause of piriformis syndrome as the repetitive action fatigues the muscle. However, sufferers often feel discomfort sitting at a desk or in a car rather than on a run. The piriformis itself may be targeted in stretches, but strength work on the surrounding hip muscles will also relieve some of the load during a run.

SACROILIAC SYNDROME

Part of the pelvis, the sacroiliac (SI) joints are located below the waist (two dimples are visible) and are the small, tight joints in the pelvis. They provide support and stability and play a major role in absorbing impact when running. SI pain occurs when the joint becomes stiff or loose. The hip or lower back can feel tight or twisted and pain is felt in the lower back and buttock, but may spread to the lower hip, groin or upper thigh.

During running, the pelvis absorbs the shock and load from the legs. If the muscles of the hip, spine and pelvis are not providing enough stability, the SI joint can become affected. There is much debate about the SI joint, a tightly packed flat joint where discussion centres around whether there is any movement in it at all. The true answer is that it cannot go from 'here' to 'there' and cannot be 'out' or 'in', it simply 'is'. That said, it can be dysfunctional and given that it is a joint and not a fixed piece of bone, optimising the joint through treatment has an incredibly positive effect on my clients.

> "Prevention of hamstring injuries is helped by increasing intermuscular co-ordination, strengthening of the glutes and enabling the hip muscles to exert pelvic control"

GROIN STRAIN

The groin is not a muscle, but the area between the abdomen and the thigh. It is the origin (tendon attachment) of the adductor muscles that serve to pull the legs inwards. These muscles are not prime movers in the running cycle so are not commonly injured by running, but they can be strained by sudden stops, starts or changes of direction. Also, runners swapping to other sports such as football can come unstuck when their comparatively weak adductors are called upon more often.

Groin strain, ranging from a dull ache to a sharp pain, is felt in the inner thigh, especially when moving the leg, and can take anything from a week to three or four months to recover fully. The principal areas to strengthen to reduce risk of injury to the adductors include the inner thigh muscles and the lateral hip muscles – especially the glutes – while core stability and balance work will also help.

LOWER BACK PAIN

The back is supported by a large, complex group of lower back muscles that support the spine, including the extensor, flexor and oblique muscles. It's unlikely that your daily routine demands the same of these muscles as running does and so you may find yourself naturally weak in this area. It is thought that approximately 80 per cent of the population will have a significant lower back pain issue during their lifetime. Although lower back pain has so many causes and contributing factors, many of them can be related to a weakness of the muscles that surround your back. Strengthening hamstrings, glutes, abdominals, external obliques and other core muscles can all increase stability and relieve stress on the lower back. I see so many runners suffering with back pain and very often this can be attributed to tight hip flexors. You can find out more on the anatomy of this area on pp. 48–9.

Symptoms of lower back pain can range from sharp localised pain through to a diffuse, widespread ache. Aside from a tightening or spasm of the muscles surrounding the spine, problems in the vertebrae and discs of the spine itself are sometimes a source of the pain. However, talk of wear and tear on the discs, 'bulging' or slipped discs is becoming a thing of the past. Changes in the spinal vertebrae can be a natural result of ageing, yet while we accept that our hair might turn grey, or wrinkles appear on our face, the notion that internally something may also show some signs of ageing worries people and can result in them going under the knife. It might be that the disc issue isn't actually the cause of the pain – and the surgery itself may cause pain, and not actually resolve the issue. I believe that some back surgery would be avoidable if these natural changes in the discs (incidences that often do not cause any pain at all) were understood and explained properly. In many cases, lower back pain sufferers can perform some simple, yet effective exercises to strengthen their musculoskeletal system and become symptom-free. If you want to remain strong or gain strength in these areas to reduce pain, then this book has some great exercises.

UPPER BACK PAIN

The slouch – a posture perfected by hours of desk work – can play havoc with the vertebrae and back muscles. Weakness can lead to a dropping of the head forwards and an outward curve in the spine when running, which in turn brings stress and pain to the upper back. While improvement in posture will help, the key is improving upper body strength, especially the trapezius and rhomboid muscles in the neck, shoulders and back and the core muscles. Standing tall enables better lung capacity and shock absorbency within the spine and is recommended.

SHOULDER AND NECK PAIN

Most runners' shoulder and neck pain injuries can be put down to form. As fatigue sets in, the chin juts forwards and the shoulders are rounded and shrugged. This puts stress on the muscles in the shoulder and at the base of the neck, which can result in nagging pains. In addition, these areas are also vulnerable to referred pain – pain felt in a part of the body other than its actual source.

The key muscles in these cases include the trapezius muscles each side of the centre of the upper back (the thoracic spine), which provide flexibility in the upper and middle spine and are often the source of referred pain; and the shoulder rotator cuff muscles, which sustain the swinging motion of the arms.

TENSION HEADACHES

Sometimes described as exertional headaches, these are a pulsating pain (rather than a sharp pain) on either side of the head. The pain can last from a few minutes to a couple of days. They may be due to dehydration or blood flow, but can also be caused by tension in the neck, shoulders and spine. The muscular issues mentioned are therefore relevant, but attention should also be paid to strength imbalances in the sets of muscles that hold the head straight, namely the extensor and flexor muscles.

> **"Talk of wear and tear on the discs, 'bulging' or slipped discs is becoming a thing of the past"**

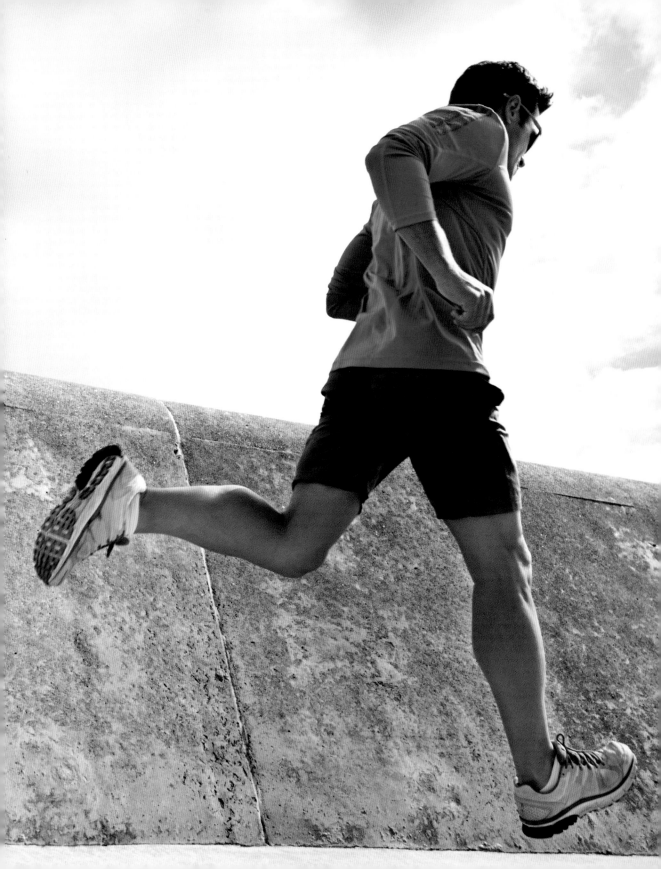

CHAPTER 11

COPING WITH INJURY

Did you know that when an athlete becomes injured they experience the same emotions as people following bereavement!? This may be hard to conceptualise for many I am sure, but if your entire raison d'être is centred around a specific competitive goal, then that is, in many cases, an obsession that goes far beyond anything else in your life. To have that taken away as suddenly as losing someone close to you can, whatever your thoughts on the subject, lead to depression.

Of course, depression is an extreme example, but I see these traits in my physiotherapy clinic all the time and not just in elite athletes – they are also experienced by competitive club runners and frankly, anyone who has attached a great deal of meaning to their running speed.

What we need here is a dose of reality. This is very much a 'first world problem'. It's not like an injured athlete is about to breach the trenches and advance over no man's land to almost certain death. What you have is a fitness goal, perhaps an event for which you're raising money for charity, and to which all your friends and family have contributed. You, and they, may also have booked travel and accommodation and, as far as you are concerned, it is impossible to drop out. The anxiety that this can produce is palpable in the clinic space where I operate. Runners do not want to be told they can't run and rarely do I utter those most heinous of words for that very reason. That is not to say that I do not need to at times, but actually all these words do is present a problem, seemingly without solution. So, just as injury will occur, an answer is also largely available.

Let me diverge for a second. Why do you buy a drill? You know those things that are loud, create dust and, at least when I'm using them, cause damage to walls. The reason you want a drill has nothing to do with wanting a drill per se, but it has everything to do with wanting a hole in a wall. What you want is the end product and if someone told you that the same accurate hole could be created by an iguana, then that is what you would buy. The only reason you have any attachment to the drill is because it will enable you to achieve your goal. Being a physio is just the same. We are the drill, not the hole. This analogy leads us to the point: a physio telling you that you cannot run is as good as a drill (or iguana) that won't create a hole. The only reason you attend my clinic is because you have issues that mean you cannot run as you would like. It's therefore my job to fix that.

So, when you attend my clinic, to assess the situation I need the answers to three key questions:

1 **What are the three things you are unable to do as a result of your issue/pain/injury?**

2 **What are your three goals once the injury is resolved?**

3 **What is it going to mean to you to achieve these goals?**

This provides me with information about what type of hole in the wall is needed, where and when you want it, and your level of desire to get it done in a timely manner.

Why do I need this information? Because without it I may provide you with a totally unrealistic treatment plan. There are always many different ways to fix an injury. In private practice this can have an effect on the cost, both financially and in terms of time. It can be very advantageous to attend more than once per week, but if the client is really not fussed about the time it will take to get better then we can take the recovery at a slower rate. If, for example, there is a significant tendon issue then using clinically proven treatments such as shockwave therapy combined with high-powered laser can speed things up by 40 per cent or more, but these require significant financial outlay. That is not to say that the desperate and time-constrained get charged more, it is just that while we have a whole host of things we can use, our company's ethos is to try to practise in the most cost-efficient way for our clients, while being as focused on their goals as they are.

So, first of all, we need to take the injured athlete to a place where they understand that their goal is of paramount importance to us. In short, we share some of the burden. Second, we do not offer road blocks, but explain what 'needs' to be done, what 'should' be done and what 'could' be done. There is no point in saying 'you cannot run' as it causes so much angst and future issues with the client's psychology, but we can say the same thing with a positive outcome. Stay with me…

Mary comes to me and she has plantar fasciitis (also known as plantar fasciopathy). In most clinics, she would be told, 'Mary, you are unable to keep running,' whereupon Mary takes an emotional nosedive and from that point onwards is deaf to everything else you say. Her goal is over, she may never run again, even though nobody has specified whether or not this is forever or just until the injury is better again.

It is my contention that a client should be presented with a solution. So here goes... see which you would prefer.

'Mary, you are still highly likely to be able to run your marathon come the autumn and it is fantastic that you have attended physiotherapy today because we have enough time to get you to that start line having completed a strong training programme and we can feel great about it when you cross that finishing line. Now there may be a period of cross training instead of running, which will push your heart and lungs equally hard, and we can build in some strength work and technical advice so that you achieve a great time as well.'

So now what Mary hears is that her dream isn't over, that she may even go faster than she expected and someone is going to share that burden with her. Of course, immediately upon reading this, many of you will say that I have given her false hope. Not at all. I am giving her hope, but it isn't false. I expect her to get better, I have tools at my disposal such as shockwave therapy that have an 82 per cent success rate. I have literally countless numbers of clients who have overcome the same injury in less time than Mary has and very, very few who haven't. There are no guarantees in life but I would bet heavily that if she follows my programme of treatment and advice then she will prevail. What if Mary comes close but doesn't quite make it? Then you know what, we did everything we could together as a team and we will both know we tried our hardest. The worst-case scenario: Mary really does herself proud and her friends and family will most likely (I hope) donate to her charity anyway. Plus, she will undoubtedly come back to race another time once she is fully fit and well. But what doesn't happen is depression, isolation and ultimately, another would-be runner giving up, never to return.

What we say to people like Mary is more important than what we do. Getting a reputation, as I have, as someone who doesn't tell a runner not to run unless it is absolutely necessary helps a great deal with referrals, as do results.

> **"It is my contention that a client should be presented with a solution. So here goes..."**

So, make sure that if you do get injured, you first of all take stock of the situation and gain some perspective. There are other races and many other things going on in our lives that have equal need for our emotional maturity. In short, worry is a pointless emotion that doesn't achieve anything other than increasing the stress hormone in your body and I am here to tell you that this hugely reduces your ability to heal from injury.

Gain perspective, set out a plan with your physiotherapist and seek to understand how and when you are going to pop back into your chosen training schedule. To give hope to all of you out there, I have witnessed a higher number of personal bests (PBs) from people returning from a well-formulated rehabilitation plan than I have from those who have taken on an overly gruelling training programme. The ability to take stock and fix weaknesses enables a process of deconstruction to reconstruct and in almost all cases the end product is superior.

So, I can truly say that, for the committed, injury can actually make you a better, stronger and faster runner.

IDENTIFYING WEAKNESSES

As a physio, before I decide on any kind of intervention, I first identify the issues. Sometimes I'm dealing with an injured runner, sometimes with a healthy and fit runner who has hit a plateau with their training. Fixing something isn't always about finding something broken, it can be about finding a part of the chain that is suboptimal and holding back performance. Runners can apply a similar methodology to their own performance.

To go back to our earlier analogy of the bike wheel, you may not see with the naked eye that the wheel is buckled, but if you were to look at the spinning wheel head on, slowed down via a video playback, you would see unwanted movement, which would clearly be affecting its performance. Worse still, other parts might wear out faster if it is left in this state.

> "Make sure that if you do get injured, you first of all take stock of the situation and gain some perspective... Worry will reduce your ability to heal from injury"

MASSAGE

Massage is a hugely therapeutic intervention – a claim supported by varying levels of scientific proof. I do not wish to get into a big discussion about the placebo effect here, but if you walk into a clinic feeling terrible and you leave feeling amazing and run a personal best, do you care what the science naysayers have to report?

Human touch into the muscles that hurt, feel tight and seem to be holding you back, when done well and firmly and in conjunction with stretching and strengthening exercises, can ward off so many aches and pains for the modern athlete. Massage stimulates blood flow and kneads away at trigger points and muscle knots in a way that nothing else does. Can I spend large portions of this book trying to convince you of this with amazing scientific review? No. I would be able to find studies that showed some great results and in equal measure those that showed no effect. Suffice to say, if it works for you, making you feel better and able to train again, then do it; it certainly isn't doing any harm.

What's more, for 18 years in my clinic, massage has formed the bedrock of our treatments and is an integral part of the manual therapy we use. Despite the fact that the technique comes under intense scrutiny from the pain scientists who would argue that by treating you in this way, we are confirming beliefs that something is wrong and making you reliant on our services. I can assure you, however, that watching so many happy athletes benefit over the years – witnessing the likes of Mo Farah, Paula Radcliffe and Steve Cram all benefit and go on to break records at the very top of the athletic community – matters more to me as evidence than a study looking at 28 American college athletes in their late teens that found massage offered no tangible or statistically relevant benefits. I appreciate the scientific community will rage at me for saying this, but who do you follow in your training? Mo? Paula? Or someone whose aim was to try to prove that a well-known and commonly used intervention was in fact a sham. The world of acupuncture has been under the same fire for decades and decades, but the Chinese just ignore it and continue to use a practice that predates our entire modern medicine culture in the West. This doesn't make it right, it just makes it a free world for those who want to have a treatment that at worst does no harm and at best has powers as yet undiscovered or is simply a very powerful placebo.

And as a brief endnote: why is placebo seen as such a bad thing? If someone feels better, can train again and move and race and win, then do they really care what dark unknown forces were at work that day? They just know that they accomplished something great and the sum total of the things they did to reach their goal all played a role, physically and mentally. I can tell you that drinking and smoking and staying up all night harm performance, but massage will not. So if it works for you, stop thinking too much and use it at will, because one day I might be able to write up scientifically what I see in clinic every day: massage works for just about everyone.

Identifying that there is an issue doesn't, however, tell you which of the 32 spokes that support the wheel is at fault. It merely tells you that there is a problem. Now you need to undertake the painstaking process of testing each of the spokes until you have a list of either loose or tight ones and then gauge how much to tighten or release each of these, followed by a retest of the system to ensure that the desired result is achieved. You then need to check everything else in the system to give the greatest possible chance of success going forwards.

As physios, however, we see patterns, which lead us to the correct 'spoke' much faster than testing every single one would. We have our own eyes and experience and lots of computer-aided technology, and artificial intelligence (AI) is starting to play a role in this area too.

But what can you do? On your own, at home or in the gym? You already have some of the answers if you listen to your body. For example, which is your stronger arm? Which leg would you rely on most, or take off from if leaping? Have you had pain or injury before? List these as carefully as you can, stating which side each was on.

FOR EXAMPLE:

1996 left knee injury

1998 left knee injured again

2000 left side lower back pain

2004 ruptured anterior cruciate ligament (ACL) on left

2005 surgery to repair ACL

2006 left side back pain

2009 left side shoulder pain

2012 neck pain and headaches started and continue.

This looks too obvious and made up to drive home a point. Actually, it is my list! You could argue that I have a clear weakness on my left side. The point is, patterns can emerge and then lead us to better diagnosis. Noting down all of these factors can really help you to start to understand your body before commencing some basic testing.

TESTING

Once you've answered the questions listed earlier, if you haven't already done so you can now go to Chapter 9 and do the tests I have laid out there. This isn't an all-encompassing physio assessment, but it will guide you to the most obvious areas to work on. For example, stand up and perform a side bend – a really strict one, with no leaning forwards or backwards and no movement at the knee or ankle, just a pure side bend. Enlist the help of a friend to place their finger at the level you can reach to with your outstretched arm, repeat on the other side, then compare the results. If one side is lower than the other, stretch the shorter side for a few days, then reassess. This should level things up, but it won't tell you what's causing it. Leave the stretching alone for a few days and then measure again. If the same difference is back again, then there is something that you do regularly that is going some way towards creating the difference. Have a good think about how you sit, your sleeping position, your desk set-up, etc and see if there are any marginal gains you can achieve through tweaking these.

If you stretch the muscle out again and your habit changes haven't made any difference, then it may be time to speak to a professional to look at this in more detail. Even if this is the case at least you now have some basic tools that you can use to perhaps help yourself.

I have a slight caveat to this, however. When someone comes to my clinic with a complex issue, it is always harder to assess them if they are partially treated, ie someone or something else (such as this book) has given them a load of exercises to do, or they have already had some treatment. This means that the usual patterns we see do not jump out so readily. The flip side, with this book's help, is that you may not need to see anyone at all. Either way, if you note down what you found and how you treated it, there should be enough information to help your physio to reverse engineer your situation.

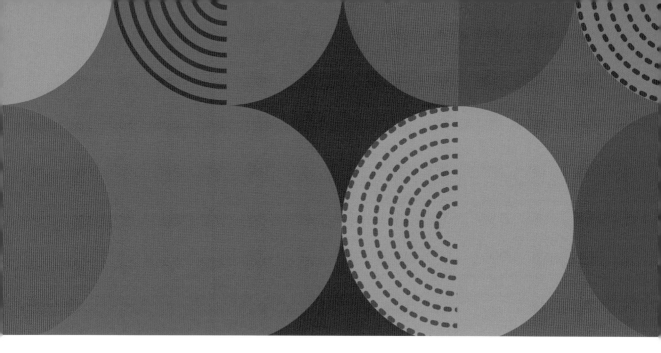

DEVELOPING A NATURAL DEFENCE AGAINST INJURY

When you find yourself in the welcome position of being injury-free and training well, your mind may well turn to the thought, 'It's going so well, I hope I don't get injured.'

This is a common position that everyone finds themselves in, so don't worry about it. It is, however, worth considering 'pain science' at this point. This is a relatively new understanding of the way our brain and pain interrelate, which is not always that helpful. The easiest way to explain it is with the term 'maranoia', which is the paranoia that comes during the last couple of weeks before a marathon (or any big race that you have been training for). The concept is simple: you start to feel that every little twinge or ache is the start of a major injury and, in many cases, start to believe that you have a race- or career-ending issue. The truth is that for the vast majority this is the mind playing tricks on you and there is nothing wrong. Consider another way of looking at it. Are you sitting down reading this? Comfortable? Perhaps you feel very comfortable. What if I were to highlight that your lower back is aching slightly, that the sit bones (ischial tuberosities) are sore and you need to adjust your position? Many of you will have just shifted slightly and suddenly become aware of an otherwise absent ache or pain, in which case you just experienced how easy it is for your conscious brain to create pain. Pain and damage are not linked. Pain is the brain's way of making sense of a multitude of signals coming back to it, then applying your personal up or down regulation to that message. Your history of injury, your beliefs, your experiences, everything you have read and been told all come into play and this then creates a reaction from your brain. That reaction might be a sensation of greater pain than is warranted.

Let's take another example. You walk into a heavy marble coffee table and hit your shin really hard. You shout and swear and hop around for a bit. Your brain, on seeing no blood or immediate swelling, had credible evidence that walking into a coffee table is hardly life-threatening and soon the pain subsides. Sure, there is a bruise over the next few days and maybe a little bump in the bone, but life continues after a few minutes of embarrassed hopping about. Now let's take the exact same injury, but this time you get it as you are crossing a road when a car, moving quite slowly, bumps your shin. Passers-by rush over, you are told to lie on the ground, a blanket is put over you, paramedics arrive and stretcher you to the hospital, X-rays and so on ensue and after four or five hours you return home with the insurance details of the driver in hand ready to make a claim. You may be advised to walk with crutches, take time off work and everyone is looking after you because you were 'run over'. The exact same injury to the tissues results in a massive increase in pain and future feelings of weakness and irritability caused by that time you were 'mown down' on a dangerous crossing.

How does understanding pain science help us ward off injury? The concept is that we have to provide ourselves with a healthy dose of pragmatism when it comes to aches and pains. Movement is often the best therapy and so spending time worrying about a potential ache or pain could in fact turn into a self-fulfilling prophecy. So my advice is to spend time making yourself as bullet-proof as possible. Give your brain so much credible evidence that you are the antithesis of injury prone by committing time to a really comprehensive strength and conditioning programme that when an actual injury strikes, you have so little to do in terms of rebuilding yourself that you spring back very quickly and minimise your time out.

All you need to do is keep teaching your body and your brain that you are not made of glass and that, with all this hard work, those aches and pains are weakness leaving the body following a hard training session and not the Armageddon your subconscious brain wants to believe them to be.

"Spending time worrying about a potential ache or pain could in fact turn into a self-fulfilling prophecy"

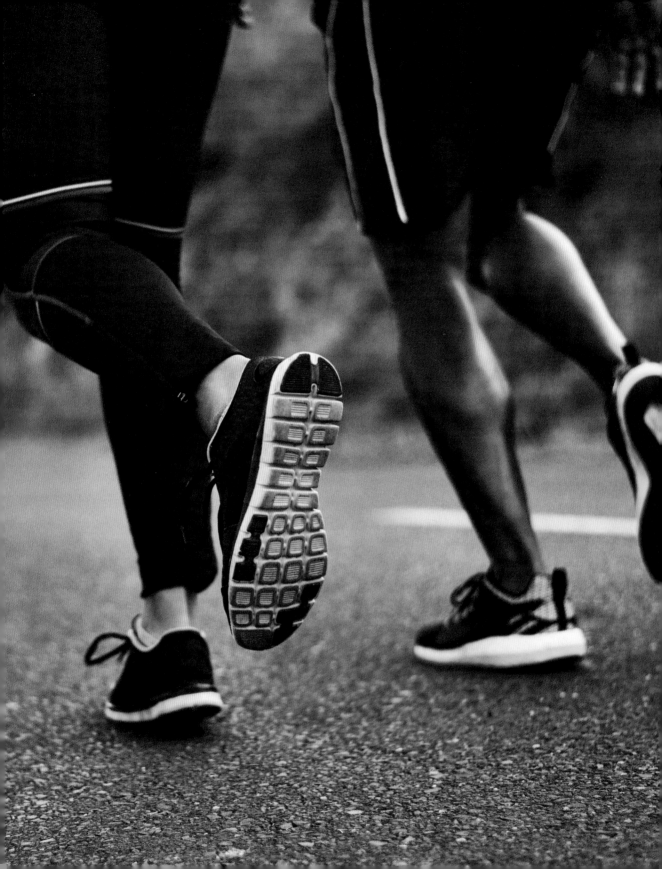

CHAPTER 12

THE BASICS

Gone are the days of languidly performing a couple of static stretches before the start of a run, or any exercise for that matter; now, the science points to one form of warm-up: dynamic exercise. Dynamic because it has plenty of movement – graduating movement, which brings each joint and muscle through its range of movement, preparing it gradually for the demands of the exercise.

In the quest for a better running technique, faster times and reduced injury risk, the warm-up is vitally important. However, the information that has been presented over the last 20 years has been conflicting and so it needs some clarification. This section provides this for you, as well as giving recommendations for ways to personalise your own version.

HOW TO USE THIS CHAPTER

The aim of this book is to help you find the best version of 'you' so that you can improve your running and stay injury-free. The basic exercises are the bedrock of this and so the finer points of how to do them properly are the primary focus of this section.

To this end, each exercise moves through an overview, the technique itself and the way it should feel, all of which are accompanied by details of the number of repetitions and sets that should be done by a beginner-, intermediate- and advanced-level runner.

But what does this mean? Who is at advanced level? The definition has nothing to do with your ability as a runner – that would be a foolish mistake to make. For example, you might be a total newcomer to running, but have had a career in gymnastics or dance, in which case you'd do the advanced level for all of the stretching exercises, but may need to do the intermediate-level strength exercises. Likewise, a regular gym-goer who takes to running may find the strength elements very easy and be able to move straight to the advanced level for those, but perhaps requires the basic-level stretching exercises. Either way, it's best to start at the beginner level to see how you get on and move on only if you can do those exercises easily and properly.

SIDE BEND

BEGINNER: two in each direction, holding for 30 seconds
INTERMEDIATE: three in each direction, holding for 45 seconds
ADVANCED: four in each direction, holding for 60 seconds

There are muscles either side of your lower back called quadratus lumborum (QL), which run from the lower ribs and attach to the upper rim of the pelvis. They stretch when you bend to the side and then contract to bring you back up again. They work to stabilise you during running and are really very important indeed. This exercise is a stretch for the QL. It's easy to visualise if you think of simply running your fingers down the outside seam of your trousers as you bend to the side. Caution is required not to lean forwards or backwards though.

Technique/exercise instructions
1 Stand with your feet hip-width apart, then run your hand down the outside of one leg and as you bend to the side, see how far you can reach down your leg.
2 Hold for at least 30 seconds. Repeat for the specified number of repetitions.

How it should feel   This is a fairly deep stretch in the side of your lower back. The release is amazing when it comes, but it could take a while to achieve any gains so perseverance is key here.

Extra advice   If you cheat and bend forwards or backwards then you'll miss the stretch altogether. Likewise, don't bend a knee or lift the heel off the floor. Where you can get to is where you are now. Work over the weeks to try and develop your range of movement. People can look like they're brilliant at this stretch, but often they are missing the key component: a straight body position.

Equipment (if required)   None.

Target area   Quadratus lumborum (QL).

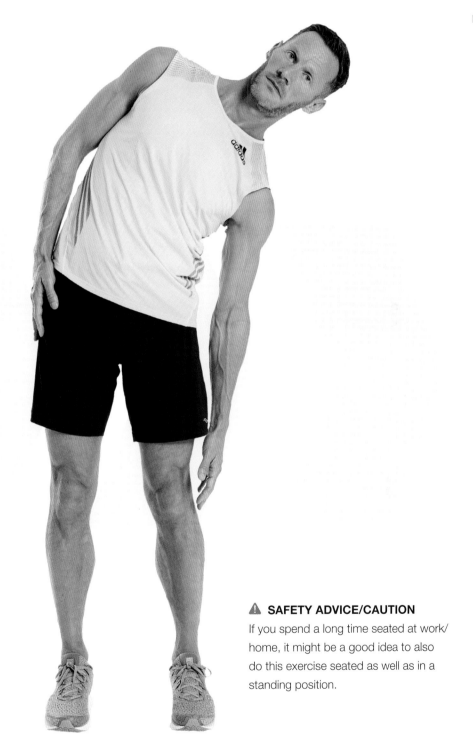

⚠ **SAFETY ADVICE/CAUTION**

If you spend a long time seated at work/ home, it might be a good idea to also do this exercise seated as well as in a standing position.

SIDEWAYS CROSSOVERS

BEGINNER: 20 repetitions with each leg
INTERMEDIATE: 30 repetitions with each leg
ADVANCED: 40 repetitions with each leg

This is a sideways jog coupled with a high knee in a line-dancing 'yee-ha' style. If you can imagine trying to go as fast as possible sideways down a very narrow corridor with occasional hurdles in your way then you can visualise this exercise perfectly.

Technique/exercise instructions

1   Moving right to left, and slowly at first, step your right leg in front of your left leg.
2   Take your right leg out into side step.
3   Lift your left leg up into a knee lift and at the same time step over and past your right leg to the front.
4   Step the right leg out to the side again and repeat. Walk it through first and gradually build up the speed and the dynamism of the movement until you are moving quite quickly to the side.
5   Come back the way you came leading with the other leg this time, ie facing the same way.
6   Repeat for the specified number of repetitions.

How it should feel   Like a flowing dance à la *Swan Lake*, just in running kit and with fewer jazz hands.

Equipment (if required)   None.

Target area   This is a full-body warm-up, targeting co-ordination, glutes, adductors and abductors.

⚠ **SAFETY ADVICE/CAUTION**   Don't trip yourself up, start slowly and build the pace. You can walk through the drill first of all and slowly build up speed. At top speed, you will cover quite a bit of distance.

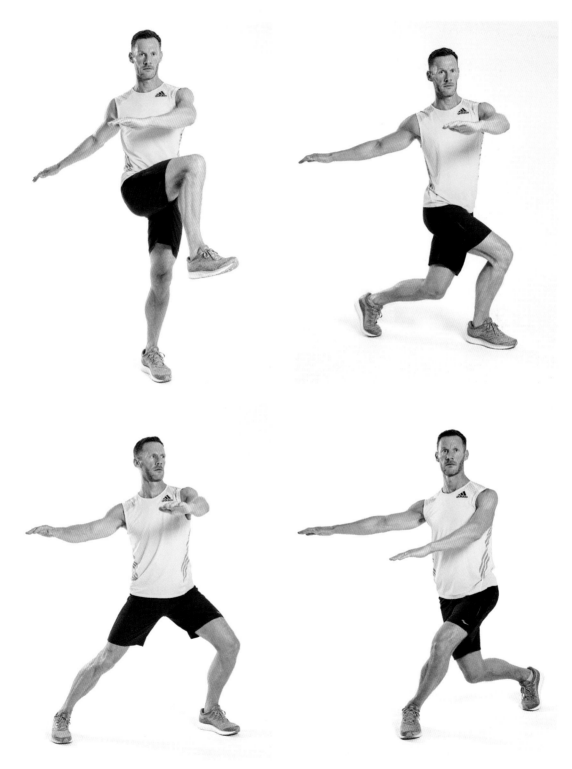

SIDE LUNGE

BEGINNER: two sets of 10 with each leg, on alternate days
INTERMEDIATE: three sets of 20 with each leg, on alternate days
ADVANCED: three sets of 30 with each leg, on alternate days

The side lunge is just like a big disco dance move by a drunk uncle at a wedding. You simply step out to the side and as you step you lower your body. There is no need to fix your tie around your head Rambo-style as per the drunk uncle, but it is important to keep control as you land and sink your hips down towards the floor, while maintaining an upright body posture.

Technique/exercise instructions
1   From a standing position, either with your hands on your hips or clasped in front of you, step out to the side.
2   When your foot makes contact with the floor, bend your knee while maintaining a good upright posture with your body. You need to drop low enough to get a 90-degree knee bend, but this may take time to achieve.
3   Start with a less acute knee bend if you cannot maintain the upright body posture and gradually build the exercise through the weeks as you get stronger.
4   Repeat for the specified number of repetitions.

How it should feel   The first few repetitions may well feel quite easy although if you have creaky knees, the sound they make may put you off a little. Knee tracking is important, so if you are concerned then see your physiotherapist for an assessment.

Over the repetitions you should start to feel some fatigue in the quadriceps and glute muscles. It is OK to progress to a fairly deep-seated burning feeling, as you would get in the gym, but only continue if you can maintain good form. There is nothing wrong with training hard, but do not sacrifice technique to squeeze out extra repetitions.

Equipment (if required)   All you need is an empty space. People performing this exercise are known to let out the odd growling noise towards the end of the set…

Target area   This is a strength exercise that will strengthen the quadriceps and glutes primarily, but a lot of ankle flexion also occurs, plus the lower back, core and hamstrings all get a good workout, too.

Did you know? The side lunge is very useful ahead of race day. When you train for running, there are few or no objects or people to get in your way. When running in a mass-participation event, such as a marathon, however, there will be a vast number of drinks bottles on the floor, people in your way and the odd rhino costume to navigate. Without this exercise, you will be hugely underprepared for all the lateral movements you will need to make and many people have suffered during longer races for this exact reason.

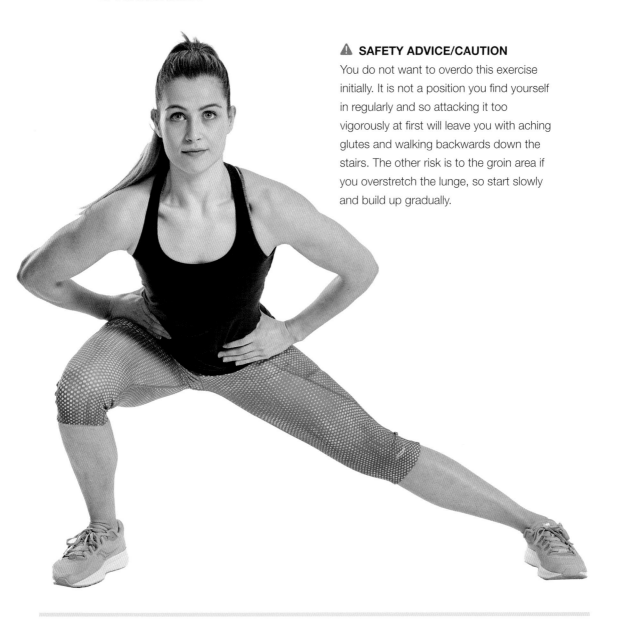

⚠ SAFETY ADVICE/CAUTION

You do not want to overdo this exercise initially. It is not a position you find yourself in regularly and so attacking it too vigorously at first will leave you with aching glutes and walking backwards down the stairs. The other risk is to the groin area if you overstretch the lunge, so start slowly and build up gradually.

LUNGE WITH KNEE HUG

BEGINNER: one set of 10 with each leg
INTERMEDIATE: two sets of 10 with each leg
ADVANCED: two sets of 20 with each leg

The lunge with knee hug is a warm-up exercise taken to extremes. You will stretch the hip flexors, glutes, hamstrings and quads all in one move while warming up the hip, knee and ankle joints. It's really very good, although it does make you look a little like you are in a Monty Python sketch.

Technique/exercise instructions

1   From standing, lift one leg up and bend the knee fully.
2   Pull the knee into your chest and then release it as you step forwards into the lunge, moving your hands to your hips.
3   As you stand up, walk forwards by repeating this with the other leg.
4   Repeat for the specified number of repetitions.

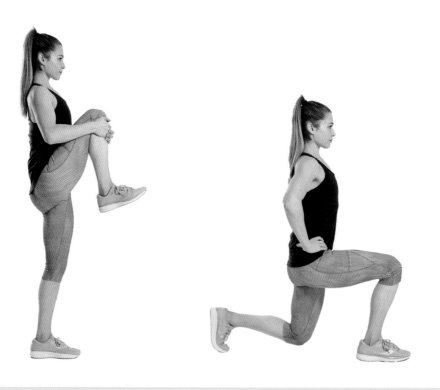

How it should feel   You will feel that you are stretching and strengthening at the same time and potentially feel like this is too aggressive for a warm-up. However, I really think you should do a few of these to get the full range of movement through your legs pre-run. The combination of stretch and strength work is simply taking you through a greater range than running will, which is a great way of preparing your body.

Extra advice   I suggest that you try this after doing some of the other, more basic warm-up movements contained within this book, such as High Knee Skips, *see* p. 118, Heel Flicks, *see* p. 119 and some hip mobility. That way you will be saving the more advanced exercises for the end of your warm-up, just before you set off.

Equipment (if required)   Just a nice clear, even surface. You will be momentarily obstructing your view of the floor with your knee, so avoid potholes or furrowed ground for this one.

Target area   Quadriceps, glutes, hamstrings, calves, lower back and core.

⚠ **SAFETY ADVICE/CAUTION**
You do not want to overdo this exercise initially. Try a few at the end of your warm-up, then build the number gradually each week until you feel comfortable. Also, be careful if it is slippery underfoot – wet grass, ice, etc – when doing this exercise.

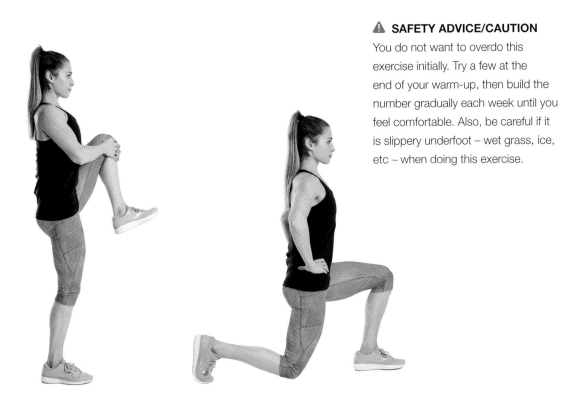

WALKING LUNGES

BEGINNER: 10 repetitions with each leg
INTERMEDIATE: 40 seconds with each leg
ADVANCED: two sets of 60 seconds with each leg

The walking lunge is a great warm-up and strengthening routine, which can be replicated on your way to work as long as you don't mind how you look or scuffs on your briefcase or bag. Also, beware of a ripping sound coming from the clothing covering your bottom if you are a skinny jeans kind of runner as stitching around this area is not done with this exercise in mind.

The exercise is, as it sounds, a large step forwards and a lunge, whereby you drop the trailing knee close to the ground with each step.

Technique/exercise instructions

1 From standing, take one large step forwards.
2 Lower the bent knee of the trailing leg towards the floor, but don't let it touch the ground. Keep your kees in good alignment and your hips level, with your head up and body straight. Move the same arm as the trailing leg in a swinging movement.
3 Rise again and bring the trailing leg through to step forwards for the second repetition on the other side. Swing the arm back behind you and swing the opposite arm up.
4 Keep walking forwards like this for the specified time or number of repetitions.

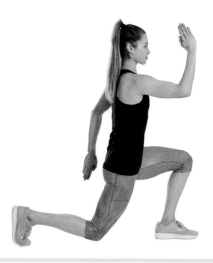
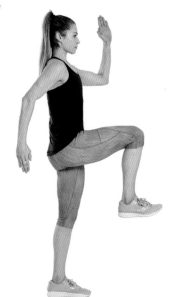

How it should feel   The walking lunge should feel like a slow and lumbering walk, similar to walking in very deep snow. The glutes should start to burn a little, as will the quadriceps.

Equipment (if required)   A reasonably long stretch of pathway or a running track are perfect for this exercise, but it can be done anywhere, including your living room, as long as you are prepared to turn as regularly as your couch demands.

Target area   This is a strength exercise that will strengthen the quadriceps and glutes primarily, but a lot of ankle flexion occurs and the lower back, core and hamstrings all get a good workout, too.

⚠ **SAFETY ADVICE/CAUTION**   It is best to do this in your trainers, making it more specific to when you run, but do not use that as an excuse to swerve this exercise at other times; it is possible to do this in just about any reasonably flat shoe or even barefoot.

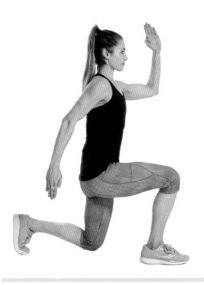

You will notice that the lunge is a popular exercise within this book. This is because it combines a number of valuable benefits, requiring balance, strength, co-ordination and flexibility, and encourages development of just about every single muscle used for running.

CLOCK LUNGE

BEGINNER: two sets of a full clock lunge with each leg on alternate days
INTERMEDIATE: three sets of a full clock lunge with each leg on alternate days
ADVANCED: four sets of a full clock lunge with each leg on alternate days

The clock lunge is a way of developing the leg strength required for runners and it also involves a great deal of proprioception and balance work. As a bonus, it offers you the chance to develop the most amazing line-dancing skills – worth bringing out when you're forced onto the dance floor at your auntie's 70th party. It's a great option for building some extra training and finding that positive outcome from a dire situation.

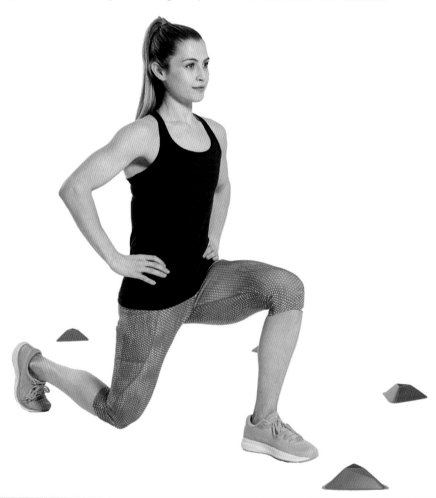

Technique/exercise instructions

1 From a standing position, complete one full lunge directly in front of you.
2 Using the same leg, turn about 30 degrees to the right and lunge again.
3 Repeat until you have performed a full circle of 12 repetitions, then start immediately with the other leg.

VARIATION: To mix this up, lunge in a variety of different directions, not taking the clock face as a sequence but making sure you hit every number once.

How it should feel The main thing is that a series of lunges is performed so do not cut back on the depth of your lunge or you will just be concentrating on the number of repetitions and direction while not maintaining the benefits of the actual exercise. A slight burning sensation in the glutes and quads is fine and shows that some good work is being done.

Equipment (if required) No equipment is needed provided you know what a clock looks like. The aim is to achieve a multidirectional exercise. If you want to branch out and do these as walking lunges with a direction change then that's fine, but you would need to be in a sports hall or park to have access to the space needed.

Target area This is a strength exercise that will strengthen the quadriceps and glutes primarily, but a lot of ankle flexion also occurs and the lower back, core and hamstrings all get a good workout, too.

⚠ **SAFETY ADVICE/CAUTION** Just be careful with your knees and ankles. If you rush this without setting up each lunge as a stand-alone exercise then you will start to develop a twist around the knee and ankle joints and this is going to cause some pain. Be more robotic about your movements and you will be fine.

> We need to increase our balance and co-ordination if we are to develop speed. Using the clock lunge is a great way to build strength at the same time.

SINGLE-LEG DEADLIFT

BEGINNER: one set of 10 with each leg
INTERMEDIATE: two sets of 10 with each leg
ADVANCED: two to three sets of 20 with each leg

The single-leg deadlift combines balance, glute strength, hip extension and core stability. It is a great functional exercise for strengthening your running and running posture. If you were to do just one exercise for your running, this would be one of the top choices.

Technique/exercise instructions

1   Stand on one leg, slightly bend the supporting knee and lean forwards, keeping good balance. Lengthen the back leg straight out behind you, keeping the hips level.
2   See if you can lower your hands below your knee and then use the glute muscle to bring yourself back up to standing.
3   Repeat for the specified number of repetitions with each leg. If you're feeling confident and fancy an extra challenge, you can add in a 1–2kg kettlebell. If you do this (pictured) you may need the hand on the hip of the back leg for balance.

How it should feel   You will feel a strong workout in your glute and also a slight pull on your hamstring. You should lower down within your tolerance for these two areas as coming back up is the harder part of the movement – don't go too low for the first few repetitions and simply work on a gradual increase in the movement.

Extra advice   You shouldn't try this exercise until you have warmed up your hamstrings a little first.

Equipment (if required)   It can be a good idea to place a small object on a stool or, if you're flexible enough, on the floor for you to retrieve and put down at each repetition.

Target area   Quadriceps, glutes, hamstrings, calf, lower back and core.

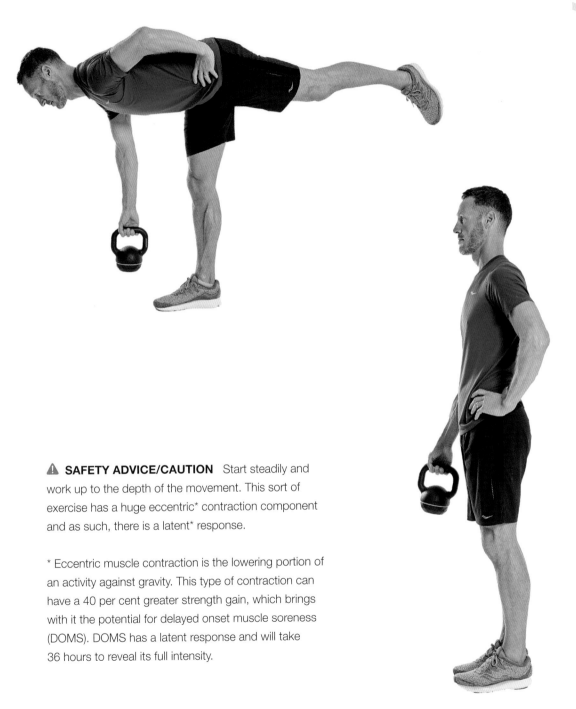

⚠ **SAFETY ADVICE/CAUTION** Start steadily and work up to the depth of the movement. This sort of exercise has a huge eccentric* contraction component and as such, there is a latent* response.

* Eccentric muscle contraction is the lowering portion of an activity against gravity. This type of contraction can have a 40 per cent greater strength gain, which brings with it the potential for delayed onset muscle soreness (DOMS). DOMS has a latent response and will take 36 hours to reveal its full intensity.

STRAIGHT-LEG LATERAL SWING

BEGINNER: one set of 10 with each leg
INTERMEDIATE: two sets of 10 with each leg
ADVANCED: two to three sets of 20 with each leg

The straight-leg lateral swing is a warm-up exercise for the abductors (smaller glute muscles) and a control for the adductors on the inner thigh. It is great for hip mobility out to the side and when brought across the midline at the end of each repetition will develop hip mobility into adduction.

The hip gets quite a lot of mobility into flexion and extension through running, so this is a key exercise for developing two more key planes of movement.

Think of a ballet dancer at the barre warming up and you won't be too far wrong (the tutu is optional, except on Thursdays when it becomes mandatory...).

Technique/exercise instructions

1 Stand on one leg and slightly bend the supporting knee. With one hand, take hold of a rail or maintain balance with a partner or wall.
2 Take your leg out to the side as far as hip abduction will allow in a swinging motion.
3 Reverse the action to return the leg downwards, allowing the leg to swing slightly past the standing leg.
4 Repeat in a swinging pendulum motion back and forth for the specified number of sets.

How it should feel   The inner thigh/groin area will feel a gentle stretch at the end range of the movement, but otherwise this should be a fairly free-flowing movement that doesn't cause discomfort or overstretch.

Equipment (if required)   A ballet-style wall barre is perfect, but frankly, any wall, desk top or a friend's shoulder will suffice. As mentioned, on Thursdays, a pink frilly tutu is required.

Target area   Adductor muscle and hip joint mobility are the main focus of this exercise.

⚠ **SAFETY ADVICE/CAUTION**   Simply start slowly and build both height and speed gradually. Do not ever seek to do this exercise at any great speed, a slow pendulum is perfect. There is always a chance that you will overdo this sort of range of movement exercise if you try to prove a point to yourself or others. Holding back is the key feature here, only increasing range when you feel it is going to be pain-free and well within your flexibility on any given day (this varies from day to day).

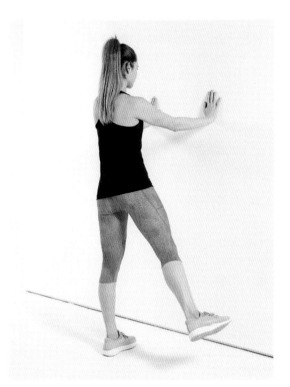 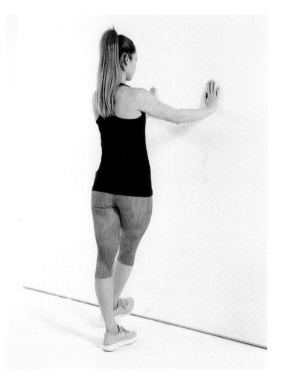

Gradually increase your range of movement each time you do this, starting without any stretch sensation and building gradually through the repetitions. Starting out too vigorously will only pull the muscles more than you want and will not give you the benefits you seek as part of your warm-up.

BENT-KNEE LATERAL SWING

BEGINNER: one set of 10 with each leg
INTERMEDIATE: two sets of 10 with each leg
ADVANCED: two to three sets of 20 with each leg

The bent-knee lateral swing is different to the straight-leg lateral swing in that it is using a short lever instead of a long one. In that respect, it can be seen as a prelude to the straight-leg lateral swing. However, this exercise does by its nature provide a little more rotation through the hip than the pure straight-leg swing and is closer to a standing clam (*see* p. 171).

It's a great warm-up exercise for the abductors and a control for the adductors on the inner thigh.

Technique/exercise instructions

1 Stand on one leg and slightly bend the supporting knee. With one hand, take hold of a rail, or maintain balance with a partner or wall.
2 Take your other leg out to the side with the knee bent to 90 degrees.
3 Lift the bent leg outwards to the side and lower under control. Unlike the straight-leg version on the previous pages, this is less of a swinging motion and is more controlled through the range, stopping as the two thighs meet again at the midline.
4 Repeat for the specified number of repetitions.

How it should feel   The inner thigh/groin area will feel a gentle stretch at the end range of the movement, but otherwise this should be a fairly free-flowing movement that doesn't cause discomfort or overstretch.

Extra advice   Gradually build your range of movement each time you do this, starting without any stretch sensation and building gradually through the repetitions. Starting out too vigorously will only pull the muscles more than you want and will not give you the benefits you seek as part of your warm-up.

Equipment (if required)   Just a partner (or wall) for balance. You don't need to be particularly familiar with the person you use, but always ask first or it gets weird.

Target area   The adductor muscles and hip joint are the main focus of this exercise.

⚠ **SAFETY ADVICE/CAUTION**

Simply start slowly and build height, but do not ever seek to do this at any great speed: a slow pendulum is perfect.

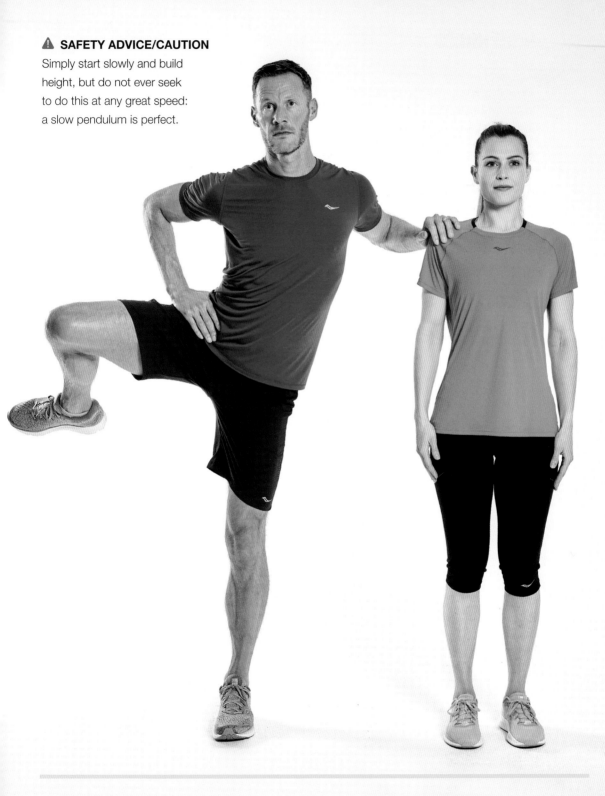

HIGH KNEES

BEGINNER: two sets of 20 seconds
INTERMEDIATE: two sets of 30 seconds
ADVANCED: two sets of 45 seconds

High knees is an exercise frequently found on a football or rugby training ground. It involves fast-cadence lifting of the knees as high as the chest area with little or no forward movement.

It's a great way to increase knee lift when running and to prepare your glutes, hamstrings, hip flexors and calf muscles for your run. Think of yourself as climbing an invisible ladder as fast as you can; doing so may give you a giggle next time you try it.

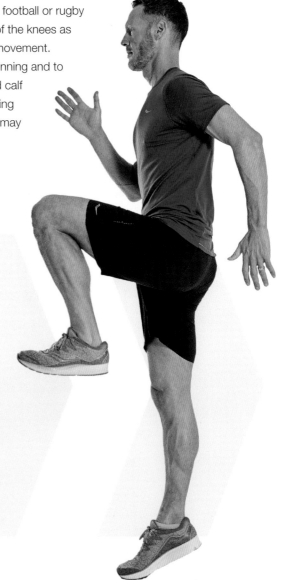

Technique/exercise instructions

1   Start by jogging gently on the spot, with your arms by your sides.
2   Gradually increase the speed and the height of your knees, bringing them up towards your chest. Continue for the specified number of sets.

VARIATION: An alternative is to tuck your elbows in to your sides and bend them so your forearms extend in front of you with flat, downward-facing palms. Now lift the knees to tap your hands each time.

How it should feel   Like a fast high-knee drill that raises the heart rate and makes any part of your body with a life of its own jump around uncontrollably.

Extra advice   Gradually build your range of movement each time you do this; you can also build up speed over the weeks. Starting out too vigorously only stresses the muscles more than you want and will not give you the benefits you seek as part of your warm-up.

Equipment (if required)
No equipment is needed although a full-length mirror will give you an appreciation of what your fellow running mates will see and bring a smile to your face, which is important for enjoying your exercise sessions.

Target area
Almost the whole body, although the focus is the hip flexors, hip joints and hamstrings.

⚠ SAFETY ADVICE/CAUTION
Beginning with the hands in place as a target at hip height is a great start. Be careful with fragile calf muscles or a recent lower limb injury. Seek medical advice if unsure.

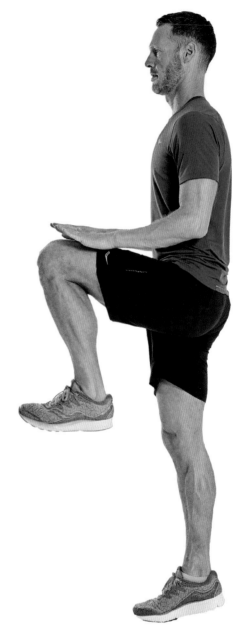

HIGH-KNEE SKIPS

BEGINNER: two sets of 20 seconds
INTERMEDIATE: three sets of 30 seconds
ADVANCED: three sets of 45 seconds

This is a bit like skipping but requires more co-ordination. In fact, getting the co-ordination right is a major part of the benefit of the exercise so try not to give up too quickly: it is a challenge. However, if you can grasp three exercises – hopping, high knees and skipping – in one, you'll have this nailed.

Technique/exercise instructions

1 Skip on the spot by hopping on your right leg while bringing the left knee up towards your chest. Engage your abs as the knee comes towards your chest.
2 Switch legs and keep skipping while pumping your arms.
3 Repeat for the specified number of repetitions.

How it should feel   Eventually, it will feel like a running drill, part of your warm-up that really gets the heart going and makes you feel explosive. In the beginning, though, it will feel like trying to pat your head and rub your stomach at the same time. It is nevertheless less frustrating than golf…

Extra advice   Start by doing one leg for several repetitions, then switch sides. Gradually reduce the number you do with each leg before you switch as you progress to expert level.

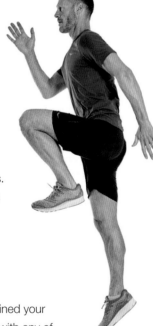

Equipment (if required)   In the early days a room without windows or cameras. When starting out on this exercise you need to be as far away from Instagram as possible… Once you've mastered it, though, make it your profile video.

Target area   This works the whole body, but co-ordination and speed of movement are the key benefits.

⚠ **SAFETY ADVICE/CAUTION**   I wouldn't start doing this if you recently sprained your ankle or have a painful knee or hip, but assuming you wouldn't really be running with any of these ailments anyway, you are good to go.

HEEL FLICKS

BEGINNER: two sets of 20 seconds
INTERMEDIATE: two sets of 30 seconds
ADVANCED: two sets of 45 seconds

Heel flicks are a great favourite for the team sports clubs. Place your hands behind you on your glutes with your palms facing outwards and without moving forwards very fast, if at all, flick your heels up until you feel them hit your hands.

This is a fantastic exercise for the workout facial expression. It has similarities with the old 80s shows that played videos of kids on a roller coaster, often trying to eat… Note to self: don't eat at the same time. Trust me, it's not a strong look.

Technique/exercise instructions

1 Start by jogging gently on the spot.
2 Place your hands on your glutes with the palms facing outwards.
3 Repeatedly flick your heels up to meet your backside and allow yourself to slowly drift forwards.
4 Repeat for the specified number of sets.

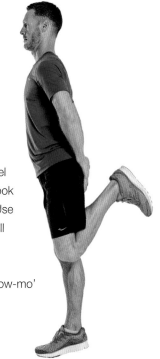

How it should feel   It feels like a technique drill for which you are trying to develop the height of the lift of your foot at the back of your stride.

Extra advice   If you watch any great runner, you will see just how high their heel comes up in the running gait. By contrast, a large number of non-elite runners look like they are scared to separate their feet from the ground and adopt a shuffle. Use this warm-up exercise in your pre-run routine and within a few weeks you too will have the heel lift of Mo Farah.

Equipment (if required)   No equipment is needed, but a camera set up on 'slow-mo' mode will give you a laugh after your session.

Target area   The glutes, hamstrings and knee joints.

⚠ **SAFETY ADVICE/CAUTION**   Be careful with your knees. If they sound like microwave popcorn cooking when you take to the stairs, start with a half range of movement.

BUTT KICKS IN PUSH-UP POSITION

BEGINNER: 10 repetitions on each side
INTERMEDIATE: 20 repetitions on each side
ADVANCED: 30 repetitions on each side

This is a strength and co-ordination exercise aimed at controlling body position and posture and having a stable core, while your trailing leg completes a cycle with a high heel lift. Too many runners 'shuffle'; use this exercise to develop range in your stride.

Technique/exercise instructions

1 Start in a press-up position.
2 Lift one foot off the floor and try to kick your butt.
3 Switch legs and repeat for the specified number of repetitions. Try to control any desire to roll the body from side to side, or to move anything other than the leg. Think of this as more of a straight-arm plank than a press-up.

How it should feel   You should feel your shoulders working to support you, but not excessively. Your core should feel fully engaged and may well be the limiting factor in this exercise. The work required to flick your butt with your heels is minimal in comparison to the core and shoulder work.

Equipment (if required)   A mat is helpful for under the hands; you could be there for a while.

Target area   Shoulders, core, quadriceps, glutes and lower back.

Did you know?   Posture is important. When someone tells you to relax, you will find yourself positioned in a posture you are used to. Slouching at a desk all day will start to feel comfortable, it will become the norm. Once this slouched posture has been accepted by your body and brain, it will be your go-to position. Take a golfer, for example. Their posture as they address the ball will more often than not replicate their desk posture at work. Improve your sitting posture and you'll improve your golf swing…

⚠ SAFETY ADVICE/CAUTION

As with heel flicks, the exercise is designed to assist you with a higher heel lift. However, this is the easy part of the exercise. If your core is weak then perhaps work on strength in this area for a few weeks before attempting this exercise.

Tighten the core and glutes as much as possible to provide a stable frame from which to work.

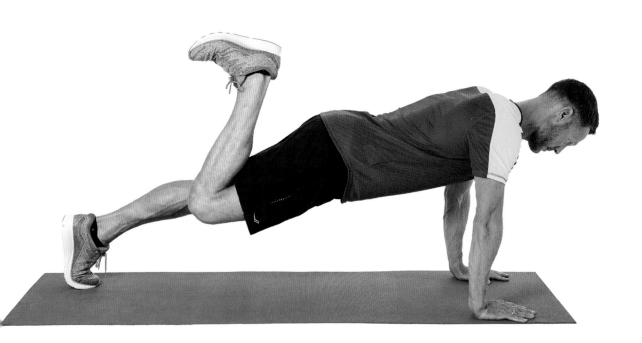

THREAD THE NEEDLE

BEGINNER: 10 repetitions on each side
INTERMEDIATE: 20 repetitions on each side
ADVANCED: 30 repetitions on each side

Start on all fours, or in a side plank (*see* p. 197) if you are already at the advanced level. There are then a few ways to do this one, the idea being to balance your core muscles while rotating the mid-thoracic spine (central spine). This adds to your available rotation, helps with breathing and is an adaptation of core work.

Technique/exercise instructions

OPTION 1:

1 Go on all fours and engage your core.
2 Take one arm off the floor and reach up as high as you can, rotating your body at the same time. Keep the other three points of contact (both knees and the other hand) on the floor.
3 Bring the hand downwards in an arc, threading it through the gap between your torso and the floor, right through until you have no more rotation to give.
4 Repeat in a continuous fluid movement for the specified number of repetitions before switching sides.

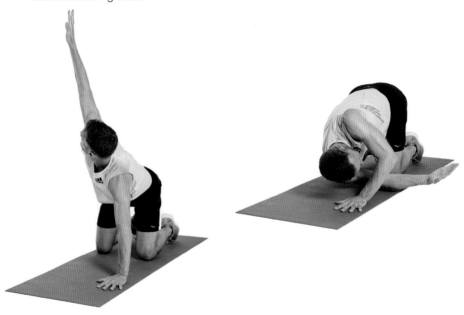

OPTION 2:

1 Start in a side plank (*see* p. 197), resting on your elbow, and thread the needle with the free hand.

OPTION 3:

1 As Option 2, but with an extended lower arm supported on your hand.

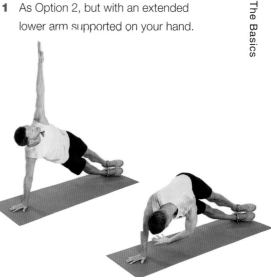

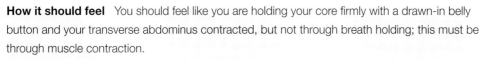

How it should feel You should feel like you are holding your core firmly with a drawn-in belly button and your transverse abdominus contracted, but not through breath holding; this must be through muscle contraction.

You will feel it's a struggle to support your weight through your shoulder and there will be a stretch through the lower back as you rotate. The mid-back won't feel like much is happening really, but rest assured, it is.

Equipment (if required) An exercise mat for your knees or hand – or at least a non-slip surface.

Target area The target is the thoracic spine, but the lumbar spine, shoulder girdle, neck and all supporting muscles are used in this exercise.

Did you know? A lot less is known about the thoracic spine (the part of the spine that articulates with the ribs) than the neck or lower back areas. Much of what we do know and how we treat it comes from an extrapolation of what we know about the lumbar and cervical spine.

⚠ **SAFETY ADVICE/CAUTION** The main issue is balance when you get to the third option. You will be putting as much work into staying in position as the exercise itself. Make sure your starting position is secure enough that you won't topple over and injure yourself later. Option 3 is advanced and requires a slow build-up.

CALF RAISE TO STRETCH

BEGINNER: 10 repetitions on each side with a 6-second stretch
INTERMEDIATE: 15 repetitions on each side with a 10-second stretch
ADVANCED: 15–20 repetitions on each side with a 12-second stretch

This is a mix of strength and stretch in one easy-to-do exercise. The calf raise is more a 'vital' than an 'important' action and should be done in isolation as well being part of this combination warm-up exercise.

The idea is to fully complete the calf warm-up by combining a stretch and strength component, which is exactly what happens when running. Calf raise, then step forwards and land in a stretch position, repeat. It's the calf version of the walking lunge (*see* pp.106–7).

Technique/exercise instructions

1 Resting your hands on your hips, balance on one leg, calf raise, then step forwards and bend the front knee to get a calf stretch on the rear leg. Move your hands to the front knee as you land.
2 Step up onto the front leg into a single-leg calf raise and then step through to stretch.
3 Repeat for the specified number of repetitions.

How it should feel The calf raise should feel like a balance exercise and not be too taxing on the strength of the muscle. The stretch should be mild but productive. Remember, this isn't directed at maximising your strength workout or replacing your calf stretching, it is an advanced and late-stage warm-up for the calf muscles.

Equipment (if required) Space and a flat surface.

Target area Gastrocnemius and soleus primarily, but hip flexors get a mild stretch as well.

Did you know? Warm-ups can feel like they last forever. I have had many jobs before, one of which was head of health and fitness for the University of Surrey in Guildford. We had many elite athletes training in the gym there who used to spend double the amount of time warming up and cooling down as they did on their main session. Quality of training is reliant on quality of preparation and recovery.

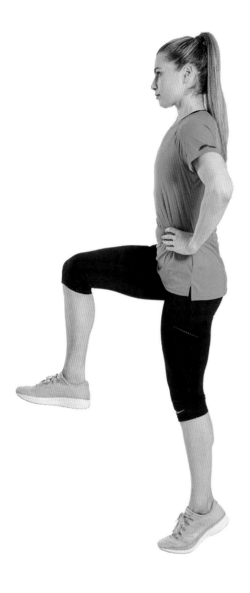

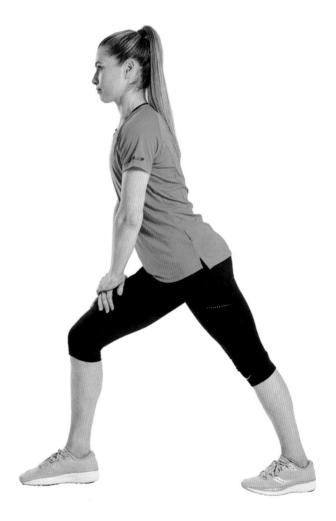

⚠ SAFETY ADVICE/CAUTION

Don't overdo this exercise. You will see that the repetitions and hold times are much lower than for a typical stretch, but this is because it is part of a warm-up routine and not to be done until you feel at least halfway to being fully prepared for the main session or event.

ARM CIRCLES

BEGINNER: 20 repetitions
INTERMEDIATE: 30 repetitions
ADVANCED: 40 repetitions

This can be done in three different ways: single arm, double arm or opposite swing directions for each arm. The idea is to increase or maintain the shoulder range of movement. Too many runners spend all their time with their arms just pumping slightly at their sides, often with a wayward elbow or two, and rarely does the left match the right side.

Technique/exercise instructions

SINGLE ARM SWINGS:

1 Rotate your arm in the biggest possible circle, aiming for the arm to brush your ear and your hip through a full circle. Change direction after you've done half the specified number of repetitions.

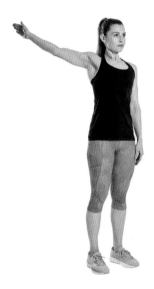

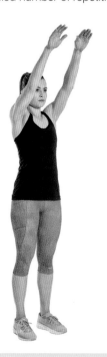

SAME-DIRECTION DOUBLE ARM SWINGS:

1 As above, but with both arms going forwards or backwards at the same time. Repeat for the specified number of repetitions.

OPPOSITE-DIRECTION DOUBLE ARM SWINGS:

1 Start with your arms by your side and begin to pendulum swing the arms back and forth in opposite directions. Gradually build up the range until they cross over by your ears and then continue to rotate full circles for the specified number of repetitions.

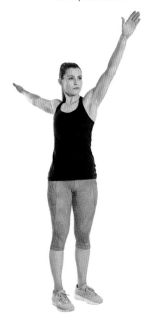
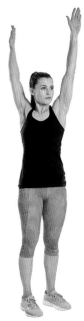
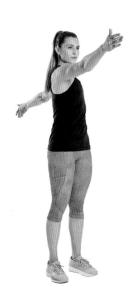

How it should feel   This should be a nice relaxing movement, with minimal stretch and some mid-body rotation that seems to ease with every repetition. The more you do this, the easier it will get and the greater you will feel as you run, with freedom of movement through your shoulders and mid-back.

Equipment (if required)   None.

Target area   Rotator cuff muscles of the shoulder, chest and upper back, deltoids and trapezius.

Did you know?   You think that running is all from the legs, but you can use your arms to set the cadence of your running. Try speeding your arms up: your legs will follow.

⚠ **SAFETY ADVICE/CAUTION**   Just don't hit anyone in the face! You really need a reversing van-style beeping noise when doing this exercise. Find space.

HIP CIRCLES

BEGINNER: 15 circles in each direction
INTERMEDIATE: 30 circles in each direction
ADVANCED: 40 circles in each direction

When a coach or training video tells you to rotate through your hips, you may find it difficult as your hips and lower back may well be stiff and tight due to the way we live our lives. You may also have an imbalance from one side to the next. Stop worrying: here we have a warm-up exercise that will enable you to get those hips moving.

Technique/exercise instructions

1　Stand with your feet hip-width apart, hands on hips and simply rotate your hips in a circle in one direction for a number of repetitions and then back the other way.
2　You will generally find that one direction is less free than the other, so repeat that side again each time you do this so it catches up. You will feel amazing after just a few weeks of commitment.

How it should feel　Like you are hula hooping your way to a 5k personal best. You could easily include said hoop in this exercise and add a bit of enjoyment/competition to the process. Can you hula in both directions?

Extra advice　Remember, this is an exercise for the pelvis, hips and trunk – it's not a back flexion and extension exercise so don't allow yourself to start leaning forwards and backwards.

Equipment (if required)　Optional pink hula hoop.

Target area　This is a full-body warm-up, targeting co-ordination, glutes, adductors, abductors and trunk.

⚠ **SAFETY ADVICE/CAUTION**　As safe as houses, nothing to worry about.

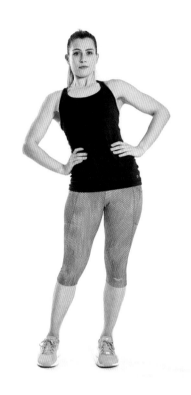
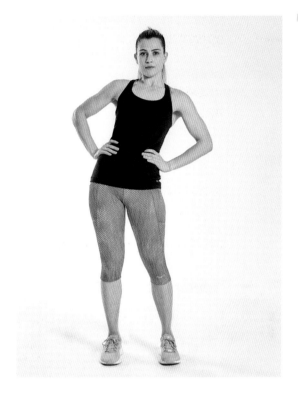
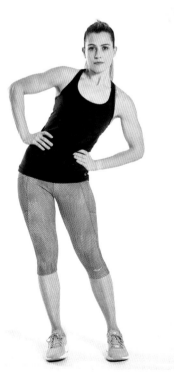
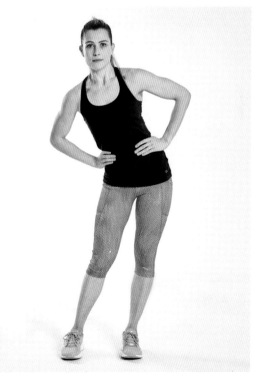

IJWTYH / UPPER BACK HALF CLOCK FACE

BEGINNER: 3-second hold in each position with five repetitions
INTERMEDIATE: 5-second hold in each position with 12 repetitions
ADVANCED: 5-second hold in each position with 20 repetitions

The letters are a reference to the shape of your arms during the exercise. Imagine yourself skydiving, face down, arms by your side, head and shoulders slightly raised. The position of your arms by your side will relate to the letters of the exercise name and held there for a period of a few seconds, arms straight down by your side would be the letter I, while arms in a crucifix would be the letter T and so on.

We do this to strengthen the shoulders, upper back, neck and lower back, all in one exercise. The benefits for posture are immense and therefore result in a better running position and performance gains for you.

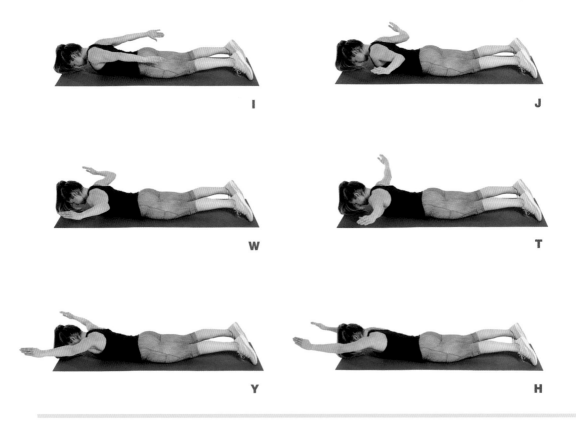

I   J

W   T

Y   H

Technique/exercise instructions

1 Lie flat on your front, arms by your sides with your head facing the floor.

2 Lift your head and shoulders up a couple of inches but keep looking at the floor (imagine you are trapping an orange under your chin).

3 Squeeze your shoulderblades together as if trying to hold a pencil between them.

4 Raise your straight arms off the ground so they remain by your sides and form the letter I and hold for the desired period.

5 Without rest, bend the elbows to 90 degrees with the knuckles facing the ceiling to make the letter J and hold this position for the desired seconds.

6 Without rest, move into the W position by abducting your arms to 45 degrees (take out to the side) – the elbow bend remains the same – and hold.

7 Straighten your arms into a crucifix position to make the letter T and hold.

8 Abduct your arms to make a Y shape and hold.

9 Move your arms straight up like a double superman to finish off with the letter H and hold.

10 Now bring your arms back down, through each letter on the way back down, holding for the same few seconds as you did on the way up.

How it should feel   Hard: this is difficult at any level. We spend too much time on computers, slouched, and looking at our phones for this exercise to be easy, but it will combat the negative effects. If it is too challenging, just hold for one second initially or break down the exercise so you do IJW one day and TYH another.

Extra advice   The key is to remain in a back extension, with the shoulder blades squeezed together, so you are setting up good posture, working the upper and lower back muscles and then really working the shoulder stabilisers at the same time. To do this well, it might be worth doing a few weeks of a basic back extension first (*see* pp. 188–9) to get that bit nailed before swinging your arms all over the place and making the exercise much harder.

Equipment (if required)   None.

Target area   Rotator cuff muscles of the shoulder, back extensors, rhomboids, posterior deltoid, deep neck flexors and extensors.

⚠ **SAFETY ADVICE/CAUTION**   If this exercise is difficult, do not push through the early weeks of introducing it too hard. You need to develop slowly and consistently to make sure that you do not cause yourself any unwanted pain from delayed onset muscle soreness (DOMS), which could feel like a bad headache through to full upper body discomfort for a few days after a hard workout.

STATIC STRETCHES

Static stretching remains the most popular and widely used form of stretching despite the fact that if you're fit and well then a dynamic warm-up is your very best option. However, there are times when a static warm-up is required. For example, if you are carrying an injury, it may be prudent to use a static stretch programme as part of your preparation instead of the more explosive dynamic version.

Static stretching is also useful as part of your cool-down, or between workouts for muscle optimisation – and the arguments for its use in those scenarios are as valid today as they have always been despite what critics may claim.

GASTROCNEMIUS MUSCLE STRETCH

BEGINNER: one 30-second stretch on each side
INTERMEDIATE: two 45-second stretches on each side
ADVANCED: two or three 60-second stretches each side

The gastrocnemius is the most superficial and therefore most obvious of the calf muscles. Divided into the medial and lateral muscles, these sit like two chicken fillets on top of the soleus muscle, which I describe as a slab of steak (sorry, vegans and vegetarians, it is just a simple, useful piece of imagery!).

Technique/exercise instructions

1   Stand facing a wall with your hands in front of you on the wall for balance. Place one foot against the wall, toes first, as high as possible, with the heel in contact with the floor at an angle of approximately 70 degrees.
2   With your hips straight and knee locked, move your whole body like a plank towards the wall until you feel a decent stretch in the calf muscle.
3   Hold for 30–60 seconds. Repeat for the specified number of repetitions.

How it should feel   This stretch is felt very easily and acutely without much effort – you do not need to drive yourself to the point of watery eyes! The recommended feeling would be a stretch that is in the region of 5–6/10 on a 0–10 pain scale.

Extra advice There are many versions of this stretch, from placing the foot behind you and leaning forwards through to dropping your heel off a step. All are valid, but I like this version as you are ultimately much more in control of the intensity and not just dropping your whole bodyweight through the muscle. It also has the added advantage of stretching the plantar fascia of the foot at the same time.

If you have a specific issue with just one of the gastrocnemius muscles, ie the medial gastrocnemius, then you could angle your foot against the wall to load the respective side more than the other. For instance, turning your foot inwards (inversion) will load the lateral gastrocnemius and turning your foot outwards (eversion) will load the slightly larger medial gastrocnemius.

Equipment (if required) A wall for your greasy handprints to adorn and maybe a step for the advanced move.

Target area Gastrocnemius muscle and ankle joint mobility.

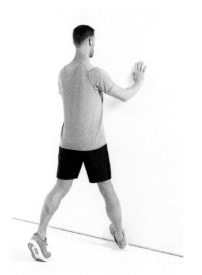
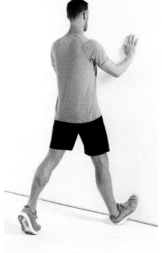
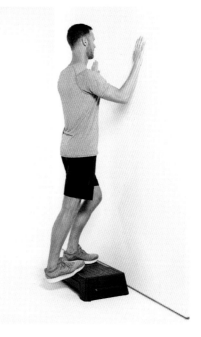

⚠ SAFETY ADVICE/CAUTION
This stretch doesn't pose any issues at all.

SOLEUS MUSCLE STRETCH

BEGINNER: one 30-second stretch on each side
INTERMEDIATE: two 45-second stretches on each side
ADVANCED: two or three 60-second stretches on each side

The soleus is the forgotten runners' muscle that sits quietly between the gastrocnemius (the muscle everyone calls the calf muscle, leaving out poor soleus) and the shin bone. Positioned underneath the more showy gastrocnemius, the flat soleus works more when the knee is bent, and the knee is bent a lot during running… Stretching the soleus is therefore, in my opinion, more important than stretching the gastrocnemius.

Technique/exercise instructions

1 Stand facing a wall with your hands in front of you on the wall for balance.
2 Bend your knees towards the wall or just one at a time (your preference if both need stretching). Keep your body upright and your heels on the floor.
3 Hold for 30–60 seconds, then repeat for the specified number of repetitions.

How it should feel This stretch doesn't feel half as satisfying as the gastrocnemius stretch; the sensation is duller, less intense. I think for this reason many clients feel they haven't actually found 'the stretch'.

Extra advice If you want to advance this stretch, then just like the gastrocnemius stretch, it can be done from a step so you can lower your heel off the edge. However, it is harder to do with a bent knee as you'll feel more discomfort in the quads than you do in the calf from the resultant isometric muscle contraction.

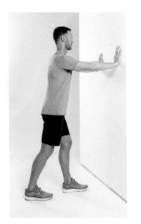
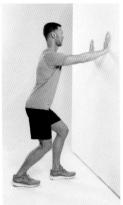

Equipment (if required) A wall and maybe a step for the advanced move.

Target area Soleus and ankle joint mobility.

⚠ **SAFETY ADVICE/CAUTION** Don't slip off the step, if you're using one. Other than this very slight potential for injury, this stretch is safer than sitting in bubble wrap in a foam room surrounded by armed guards.

SHIN PARTIAL LUNGE

BEGINNER: one 20-second stretch on each side
INTERMEDIATE: one 40-second stretch on each side
ADVANCED: two 40-second stretches on each side

The shin is a relatively understretched area except for those who work on their knees a lot, or swimmers. What we are really trying to do with this stretch is expand the angle that can be created by pointing your toes. By kneeling on a reasonably soft floor covering or mat, you will be stretching the toes out and putting pressure through the front of the ankle joint. This can cause some irritation so the shin partial lunge is a great way of isolating the muscles of the shin without causing this irritation and is ideal for those with already poor ankle range of movement (ROM).

Technique/exercise instructions

1   Stand with a wall to your side that you can use for balance if needed.
2   Imagine you are about to kick a football in a wide lunge stance, but your outstretched toes touch the floor.
3   In a slow and controlled manner bend your knees until you feel a stretch in the shin muscles. Alter the size of the lunge and the amount of knee bend to increase or decrease the amount of stretch.
4   Repeat for the specified number of repetitions.

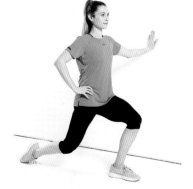

How it should feel   This stretch is harder to feel than most. It's also a balancing position, in which you need to minimise wobbling to ensure you are making the most of the stretch.

Extra advice   If you can already kneel and sit on your heels then that is an easier stretch to do since it eliminates the balancing element. Just be careful about the potential for irritation at the anterior ankle. A softer surface will reduce this irritation.

Equipment (if required)   Exercise mat.

Target area   Tibialis posterior and tibialis anterior.

⚠ **SAFETY ADVICE/CAUTION**   Just keep in mind the ankle joint irritation. You won't notice it's been unhappy until you stand back up…

QUAD STRETCH

BEGINNER: one 40-second stretch on each side
INTERMEDIATE: two 40-second stretches on each side
ADVANCED: two 60-second stretches on each side

The quadriceps are the muscles on the front of the upper leg, known commonly as 'the quads'. These are the muscles whose overuse makes you walk backwards down the stairs after running your first marathon.

This is possibly the most common of all the stretches that runners do. It's so easy: stand up and lift your heel to your backside… But wait, there are so many ways to make this stretch of more use. You've been doing it wrong all these years! Read on…

Technique/exercise instructions
There are three potential starting positions: standing, lying on your front and kneeling.

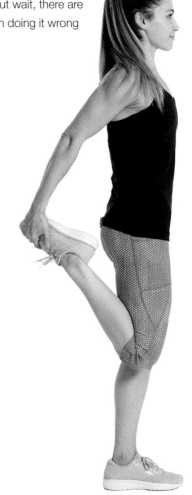

STANDING:
1 Stand with your feet hip-width apart and slightly bend one leg. Pull the foot of the other leg as far as you can towards your glutes. Ensure that your bent knee doesn't go in front of your straight leg. If you can't reach your leg, put on some old 70s flares, grab the loop of trouser at the ankle and pull that towards you. (The invention of skinny jeans may have meant that more people had to stretch their quads further. Or else everyone gave up…)
2 When in position, push your hips forward to increase the stretch. Hold for the specified time.
3 Repeat for the specified number of repetitions.

LYING ON YOUR FRONT:

1 Lie flat on your stomach on an exercise mat, then pull the foot of one leg up as far as you can towards your glutes.

2 This time, your knee will be unable to pop forwards, which means this is a true form of the stretch and there's no chance to cheat.

3 Repeat for the specified number of repetitions.

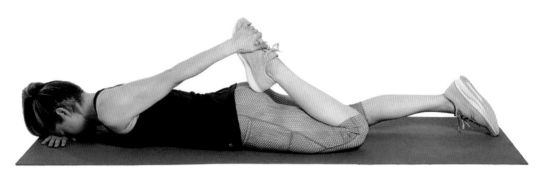

KNEELING:

1 This is only for the advanced. In a kneeling lunge (with your knee on a foam block or a pillow), reach back and pull your foot to your backside. You will be stretching the quad muscles and at the same time the hip flexor.

2 Continue for the specified number of repetitions.

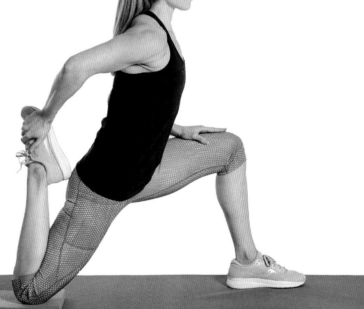

VARIATIONS:

All the quad stretches on the previous pages can be developed by choosing where to hold the foot. Taking hold of the foot centrally and pulling directly to the middle of the backside will give more of a stretch to the central quads, the rectus femoris. When you take hold of the foot around the big toe and pull the foot out to the side, you will feel the stretch more on the medial fibres of the quads, known as vastus medialis. The little toe hold, using the other hand, will bring the foot across to the other buttock and load the lateral quad muscles, known as vastus lateralis.

If you feel really confident in the kneeling version, you can try stretching both quads together as shown here. Any pain in the knees is a signal to stop immediately though.

How it should feel   The basic moves are still a deep stretch to the quads, but as you become advanced and start to stretch both the quads and the hip flexors in the kneeling position, the stretch will be quite significant. Try not to allow yourself to be in a lot of pain when stretching – mild and soothing are the buzzwords.

Equipment (if required)   Exercise mat and a foam block or a pillow for protecting the knees is quite handy.

Target area   Rectus femoris, vastus medialis, vastus lateralis, vastus intermedius, psoas major and minor, iliacus and, therefore, iliopsoas.

Did you know?   The rectus femoris (central quad muscle) is one of the few muscles that crosses two joints and so can be used as a knee extensor but also a weak hip flexor. For this reason, the kneeling stretch is far greater as it covers both joints and gives the best stretch to this muscle.

⚠ **SAFETY ADVICE/CAUTION**   Work through the stages to make sure you don't just try the kneeling stretch first; it takes a bit of getting used to.

HAMSTRING STRETCHES 1

BEGINNER: one 40-second stretch on each side
INTERMEDIATE: two 40-second stretches on each side
ADVANCED: two 60-second stretches on each side

The hamstrings are located on the back of the upper leg. They are responsible for knee flexion, but due to the fact that most runners have long and weak glute muscles, the hamstrings spend too much of their day trying to help extend the hip. This makes them tight and fatigued and more susceptible to chronic injury.

Runners need to develop some length and strength in their hamstrings in order to prevent injury to the muscles themselves, but also to the lower back, and to prevent pelvic tilt and a variety of other issues associated with muscle imbalance in this area.

The biggest issue here is that everyone wants to stretch the hamstring with a locked knee, which is ludicrous as they are basically just irritating the sciatic nerve and leaving the muscle largely untouched. Try it. Stretch a straight leg and tell me where you feel the burning pain! You will find it behind the knee, where there is no hamstring muscle at all. The hamstring muscle belly is higher up the leg. Stretching with a bent knee, holding the same knee angle and leaning forwards, however, will mean you feel the stretch right in the muscle belly – job done!

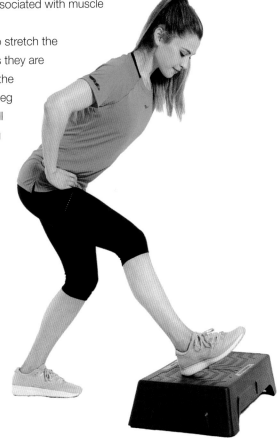

Technique/exercise instructions
STANDING:

1 Find a small box or step and put your heel on it with a bent knee. Keep your back straight and bend forwards at the waist. Hold the stretch for the specified time.

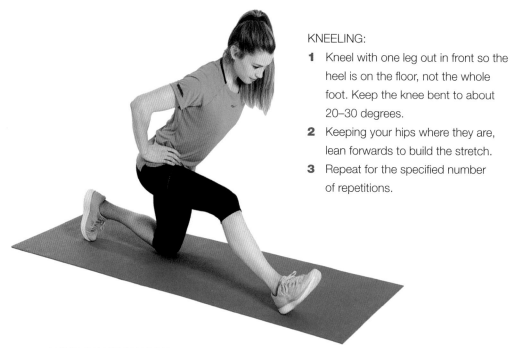

KNEELING:

1 Kneel with one leg out in front so the heel is on the floor, not the whole foot. Keep the knee bent to about 20–30 degrees.

2 Keeping your hips where they are, lean forwards to build the stretch.

3 Repeat for the specified number of repetitions.

LYING ON YOUR BACK:

1 Lie with your legs straight out in front. Lift one leg up and ask a partner to support your heel. A variation is to lie with your legs going through an open doorway. Lift one leg up and place it on the frame of the door. In both variations, the outside leg can be bent or straight.

2 Keep the knee bent as your partner lifts your heel, or the heel slides up the doorframe, until you have a nice stretch. The closer your bottom is to the base of the doorframe (if using) and in either variation the higher your foot travels towards the ceiling, the greater the stretch.

3 Continue for the specified number of repetitions.

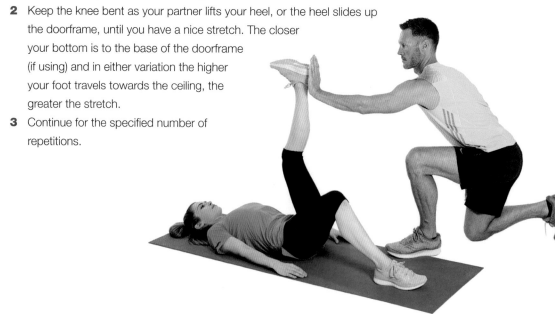

How it should feel   Hamstring stretches always feel tight and awkward to me and most non-ballet-enthused men and runners have some of the tightest hamstrings known to man (footballers' are much worse than runners' if that makes you feel better).

   This stretch can create a sickly feeling of always being a bit too much so self-regulate. Don't become competitive with anyone except yourself. Even if you are essentially unable to start the stretch much beyond 90 degrees of knee bend, don't worry: keep at it and your ability will grow faster than even you think possible.

Equipment (if required)   A step and a partner or a quiet doorway.

Target area   Biceps femoris, semitendinosus and semimembranosus.

Did you know?   Hamstrings originate from those sit bones you can feel when you perch on hard chairs. There are three hamstrings and they descend down the leg, one going to the outside and the others reaching the inside of the leg, all attaching just past the knee joint. Their relationship to the position of the pelvis is significant and hence why tight hamstrings can lead to lower back pain and postural changes, so look after them.

⚠ **SAFETY ADVICE/CAUTION**   It takes time to improve the flexibility of the hamstrings, but the early results show shortly after starting. I would suggest that after just one week of committed stretching your stride will lengthen and you will experience less stiffness in the lower back.

> Most people report having tight hamstrings,
> but also report that they know how to stretch them.
> This is the definition of madness.
> It takes one to two minutes per day,
> so come on!

HIP FLEXOR STRETCH

BEGINNER: two 30-second stretches, daily
INTERMEDIATE: three 45-second stretches, daily
ADVANCED: three 60-second stretches, daily

This is definitely a huge part of your prehab and rehab if you spend any part of the day sitting. When you sit, your hip flexor is shortened. When you run, you ask the same muscle to extend to its full length on the back swing of your leg. How many runners try to fit in a run soon after finishing work for the day, leaping from their desks to maximise their run time? Loads. Having spent around eight hours at a desk with short hip flexors, they then switch to 60 minutes of running with the expectation of a long and flexible hip flexor. It's not going to happen!

Technique/exercise instructions

1   Get yourself into a lunge position with the trailing knee resting on the floor (on a cushion or exercise mat). Make sure your front foot is further away from you than you think it should be, ensuring the knee angle is greater than 90 degrees. Keep your body upright (it's fine to rest a hand on something for balance).
2   To bring the stretch 'on', take your body forwards until the knee of the front leg reaches a 90-degree bend.
3   If you still can't feel the hip flexor stretch, rotate your body away from the trailing leg.
4   If that still doesn't do it, take your arm on the side of the trailing leg and place a hand between your shoulder blades, then lean slightly away from the trailing leg.
5   Repeat for the specified number of repetitions.

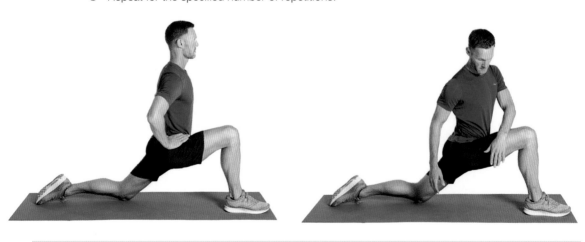

How it should feel   You should experience a mild stretch in the location of the hip flexor (the front of your hip and a little into your lower stomach).

   If you feel any discomfort in your lower back that means you are either leaning back rather than having an upright posture, or your pelvis is in anterior rotation, so tuck your hips back under your body with a little pelvic thrust thrown into the movement.

Equipment (if required)   It may be of benefit to use a fixed surface or chair back to balance on during the stretch.

Target area   Tensor fasciae latae (TFL), psoas major and minor, iliacus, iliopsoas and rectus femoris.

Did you know?   The hip flexor originates from your lower spine and travels through to the front of the hip. The hip flexor muscles are always stronger than the lower back. If you have lower back pain, it's highly likely that you have tight hip flexors. Stretch as above and watch your lower back pain disappear.

   Also, the hip flexor shares a nerve with the male testes. Pain in the testicle on the side of the tight hip flexor is not uncommon. Do not use this as a guide: always consult a GP if you experience this pain. However, your GP may not lead with the tight hip flexor diagnosis, so stretch at the same time as it may well help/be the cause.
NB: I strongly advise you see a doctor if you have a medical issue such as this as a delay in receiving an accurate diagnosis could be life-threatening.

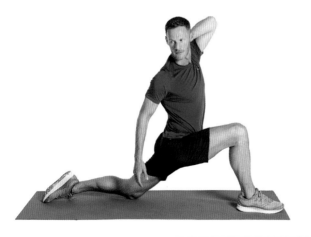

⚠ **SAFETY ADVICE/CAUTION**

Make sure you get the positioning right for you. It's OK to search for this stretch a bit. Watch your back doesn't start to hurt and if needed rest your knee on something comfortable. Just because all your running buddies can find the stretch simply by using the one position doesn't mean you will too – the position can be as individual as a glasses prescription.

TFL AND ITB STRETCH

BEGINNER: two 30-second stretches, daily
INTERMEDIATE: three 45-second stretches, daily
ADVANCED: four 60-second stretches, daily

The tensor fasciae latae (TFL) is the contractile component of the iliotibial band (ITB), which is responsible for the stability of the knee joint in motion. The ITB itself has the tensile strength of steel and cannot be stretched, hence the only place for release is the TFL. This muscle is easy to palpate by sliding a finger into the coin pocket on a normal pair of jeans.

Technique/exercise instructions

1 From standing, slide one leg backwards and around the back of the other, until your little toes are parallel with about 30–60cm (1–2ft) between your feet.
2 Take the same arm as the back leg over the head and push the hip out laterally. Lean your body to the side of the standing leg. Place your lower hand on your hip.
3 Repeat for the specified number of repetitions then repeat on the other side.

VARIATION: If you want to increase the stretch, raise your other arm upwards, bend your elbow and slide your hand down between your shoulder blades. Now, try to push the back leg hip forwards and in an arc towards the standing leg (you will experience very little movement, but the stretch will intensify).

How it should feel A mild stretch in the location of the TFL.

Equipment (if required) It may be of benefit to use a fixed surface or chair back to balance on during the stretch.

Target area This stretch targets the tensor fasciae latae (TFL). While it is almost impossible to isolate one muscle during a stretch, this is the target. You will also be stretching to a lesser degree the quadratus lumborum (back side flexor), peroneal longus, biceps femoris, latissimus dorsi and lateral glutes.

Did you know? Many runners spend a long time foam rolling their ITB. The fact is, though, the ITB is no more likely to lengthen under the efforts of a foam roller than it is at the desk at which I am sitting right now. What's more, foam rolling an ITB is incredibly painful: while it has no stretch receptors, it is full of pain sensors. There may be some benefit to the surrounding fascia, but only if you want to endure the pain.

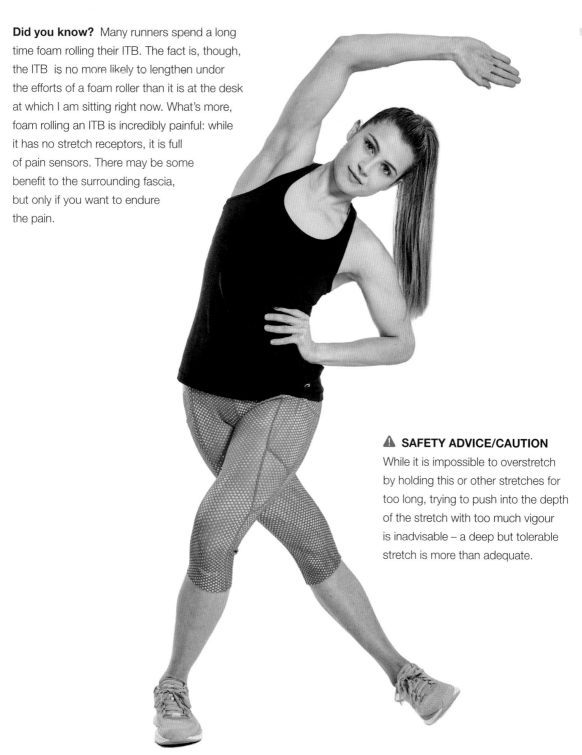

⚠ **SAFETY ADVICE/CAUTION**
While it is impossible to overstretch by holding this or other stretches for too long, trying to push into the depth of the stretch with too much vigour is inadvisable – a deep but tolerable stretch is more than adequate.

LOWER-BACK LEG HUGS

BEGINNER: one 30-second stretch on each side
INTERMEDIATE: two 30-second stretches on each side
ADVANCED: two 45-second stretches on each side

The lower back is seen as vulnerable, but in reality it is as strong as you make it. Lack of flexibility in the muscles that operate around the back, however, can lead to many issues. All around your back is an area that should benefit from great movement – side to side, forward flexion and extension, plus the myriad combinations of these we use in everyday life – for example, reaching into the back seat of a car simultaneously involves back extension, rotation and side flexion. Running, too, asks a lot from the muscles involved with lower-back rotation. This is because although you are not side flexing along the pathway (hopefully), those muscles still need to work to prevent unwanted movement.

Technique/exercise instructions

1   Lie on your back and, keeping your back flat on the floor, pull your knees towards your chest, not your head – this is not a chance to curve your back up and roll up into a ball.

2   Repeat for the specified number of repetitions.

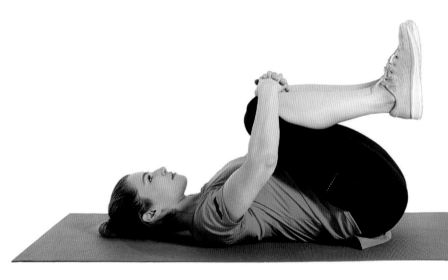

How it should feel   You should feel a lower-back stretch, plus some to the hamstrings, high up by the glutes.

Extra advice   People tend to be paranoid about their backs. This is in part down to the fact that we commonly hear about people who had X, Y or Z happen to them as a result of a bad back. As a consequence, we start to grow slightly anxious about our backs and so the slightest tweak results in us both consciously and subconsciously applying all this 'knowledge' to the situation and often creates much more pain than is reasonable. Going forwards, you will also feel that your back is vulnerable and start to hold yourself differently and, undoubtedly, move less. The less you move, the less you are able to move, and so the prophecy becomes self-fulfilling.

One way to ensure that you have (and feel like you have) a really bullet-proof back is to work hard to make sure your back is strong and maintain flexibility throughout by doing this and other back mobility exercises.

Equipment (if required)   Don't do this on a very hard or a very soft surface – an exercise mat is perfect.

Target area   Lumbar spine extensors, glutes and hip joints.

⚠ **SAFETY ADVICE/CAUTION**   There are some videos and information out there telling you that this is a bad exercise that will make your back worse. I have to say, physiotherapists do not talk about 'bulging discs' or 'damage' any more. The body will react very well to load if it is developed incrementally over time. This idea that by hugging your knees you will be pushing the spinal discs 'out' is nonsense. You are performing a movement that your skeleton is perfectly capable of doing, so long as you don't overstretch by having someone jump on top of you while you're hugging your knees.

NECK ROTATION, SIDE FLEXION AND FLEXION STRETCHES

BEGINNER: two in each direction, holding for 10 seconds
INTERMEDIATE: three in each direction, holding for 20 seconds
ADVANCED: three in each direction, holding for 30 seconds

The neck is supporting the single heaviest individual item on the human body: the head. Your neck needs you, so let's make sure you know how to look after it. This simple yet very effective set of stretches will help you do just that. The stretches involve a series of specific movements with and without resistance applied with your fingertips.

Technique/exercise instructions

NECK ROTATION:

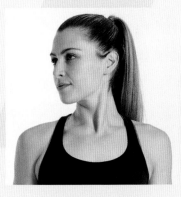

1 In a seated or standing position look over first your right shoulder and then your left – do not move your upper body or shoulders at the same time. Use a mark on the wall, for example, to gauge how far you were able to turn your head each way.

2 Now go back to that point, apply two fingers to your jaw and try to stretch your neck gently a little further. Repeat this a few times, with 10–30-second holds.

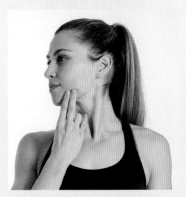

3 You can advance this performing a proprioceptive neuromuscular facilitation (PNF) on the rotation muscles. Push your head against the resistance of the fingers so there is no movement; instead, there should be an equal and opposite force from each (this doesn't need to be a strength test, 20–30 per cent of strength is perfect). Hold for eight seconds, release and then rotate your head a little further. You can repeat this a few times and literally watch the range of movement improve.

You will lose some of this mobility as you go about your daily business, so repeating the exercise three times per week will provide the best opportunity for growth.

SIDE FLEXION:

1 You then need to do the same into side flexion (dropping your ear down to your shoulder). Stand or sit, keeping your shoulders relaxed and trying to resist the temptation to lift them up.

2 Side flex your head to try and get the ear as close to your shoulder as possible.

3 Place two fingers on top of your head to the side and apply pressure downwards to develop the stretch. Repeat this a few times, with 10–30-second holds. If you want to try the PNF stretch from there then do so, but again use just 20–30 per cent of your strength.

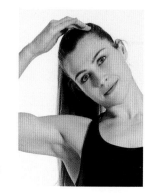

FLEXION:

1 Stand or sit, keeping your shoulders relaxed and trying to resist the temptation to lift them up.

2 Gently drop your head down towards your chest – this should be done very carefully, just to elicit a gentle stretch.

3 Place two fingers on top of your head to apply pressure downwards to develop the stretch. I would do this maybe once a week as many of us have a tendency to drop our heads forwards anyway. If this is you, work more on the other stretches instead.

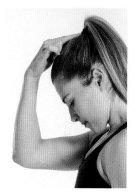

How it should feel   Movement should be gentle and not aggravating in the slightest. Go very easy with neck stretches – it doesn't need to feel like a second training session! Slowly develop the range of movement over weeks and months.

Equipment (if required) None.

Target area   Side flexors, neck extensors and neck rotators.

Did you know?   The deep neck flexors run an interesting course and attach to the cervical spine in such a way that strengthening them helps with posture. You might think strong neck flexors will pull your neck into more flexion, but actually they pull your head more on top of your shoulders. When you consider that a head weighs on average 5.4kg (12lb) and that every 2.5cm (1in) it is moved forwards adds 4.5kg (10lb), it's easy to see that the head being even just a few centimetres forward adds considerable weight. So, let's get the head back on the shoulders.

⚠ **SAFETY ADVICE/CAUTION**   Don't overdo the stretch. Try to think about neck posture and how far forwards your head is when you are on your phone, tablet or computer.

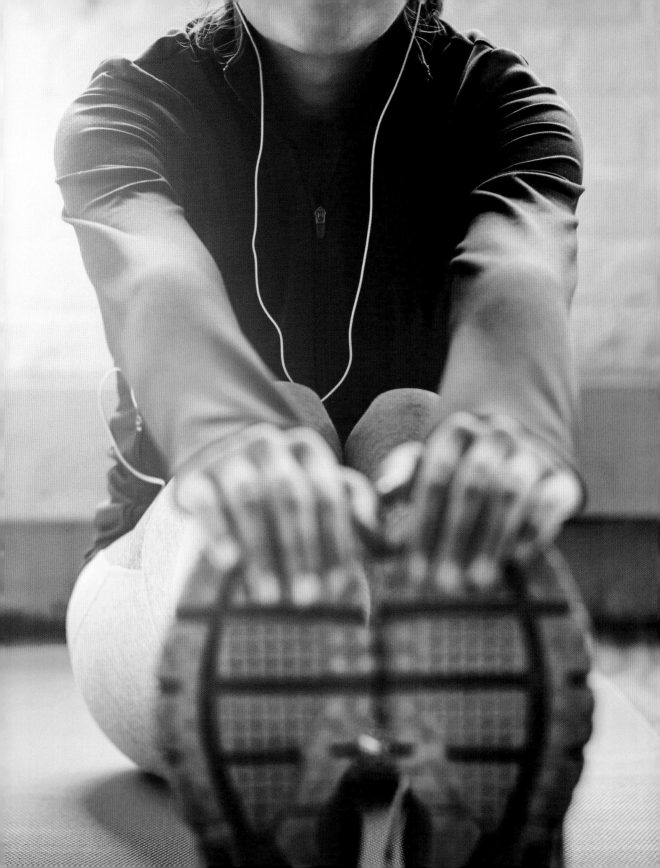

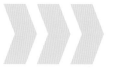

CHAPTER 13

STRETCHES AND STRENGTH EXERCISES BY BODY AREA

This section provides useful and challenging exercises ordered by body area, and is a chapter you can use as a reference point, coming back to it time and time again as you need it. There are good basic stretches, but also a variety of strength exercises that will help you build that all-important fitness for race day. For therapists, this is the section that you could use for your exercise prescription for your clients.

It's important to state up front that, while I suggest you give every exercise in this chapter a go at some point, some of these exercises will be of more use to you than others. If you're a regular runner, you'll already be aware that you have certain injury-prone areas or weaknesses that you might want to address. My intention is to help you build a regular set of stretches that you enjoy doing, customised to your needs. But there's also enough choice here that if you develop a niggle in a different part of your body, or simply get bored of repeating the same routine, you can change it up a bit.

FOOT

The foot is the anchor between you and the ground. We simply must look after this piece of equipment to enable us to both feel and respond to the ground and its reaction forces. The more able the foot, the better the runner.

TOWEL GRABBING

If you want a strong and intelligent foot then look no further. The act of dragging a towel along the floor using your toes strengthens the small muscles of the foot and begins their journey to becoming a more intelligent body part that's able to sustain your running load of the future.

Technique/exercise instructions

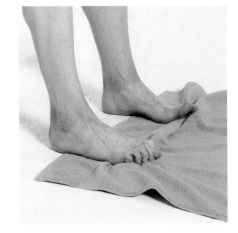

1 Find an area with a slippery surface, such as wood or tile, not carpet. Sit in a chair with a hand towel spread out neatly in front of you lengthways.

2 Place your bare feet side by side, separated by a couple of inches, with just the toes on the towel; the rest of your feet should be on the floor.

3 Imagine your heels are glued to the floor, but your feet are able to lift up (like working the accelerator on your car).

4 Now grab the towel with your toes and pull it towards you with just your feet so it scrunches up under your feet by your heels, which are still on the ground. Keep going with repetitive movements until there is no space left.

Replace the towel in the starting position and repeat the exercise. Continue for about two minutes at a time.

How it should feel Difficult at first. You may find that one foot struggles to pull the towel, or the towel just won't move. For others, the towel will glide seamlessly towards you and this will feel like a strong, controlled movement. This is where we all need to try to get to, for fully functioning feet.

Equipment (if required) A chair and a hand towel.

Target area Lumbricals, flexor digitorum brevis, flexor hallucis brevis and interossei.

⚠ SAFETY ADVICE/CAUTION

This is a highly addictive exercise and will have you seeking friends and family members whom you can persuade to try it, or you will simply be seen fidgeting with your toes, which will become irritating to those around you.

BIG TOE EXTENSION

BEGINNER: hold for 30 seconds on each side, daily

INTERMEDIATE: several holds of 60 seconds on each side, daily

ADVANCED: hold stretches for as long as you can, although the likelihood is that if you have reached this level then your big toes are already of adequate mobility and you could simply maintain the stretch by doing the beginner stretch

The big toe has a habit of losing its movement, largely due to the way we live: always in shoes and often ones that are a tighter fit around the toe box area. Working on maintaining your big toe movement can be vital for good push-off while running and reduces the risk of injuries such as plantar fasciitis.

Technique/exercise instructions

1   With bare feet, take hold of your big toe with your fingertips and pull it up towards your shin. Do this at first with a bent knee and then, if flexibility allows, you can do this with a straight leg.

2   Hold for the specified time, then repeat on the other side, making sure you do it an even number of times for each foot. Relax between sets.

How it should feel   You should feel a stretch along the base of the foot. If you have significant pain in the toe joint then you need to have this looked at in case there is an issue with the joint itself. A physio or podiatrist can help you here.

Equipment (if required)   None.

Target area   Plantar fascia.

Did you know?   So far as we know, there hasn't been a single case of bunions or associated disorders of the big toe in tribes or cultures where feet haven't ever been enclosed in shoes.

⚠ **SAFETY ADVICE/CAUTION**   If you have a significant bunion or hallux valgus (where the big toe is moving into the other toes) then seek advice from a health professional before doing this exercise.

ARCH BUILDING

BEGINNER: one set of 5–10 repetitions
INTERMEDIATE: two sets of 10–15 repetitions
ADVANCED: three sets of 20 repetitions

In order to develop the natural arch in your foot, or at least the strength within the foot, you can work on lifting and slowly lowering your arches when standing. This makes you look a little like a short person trying to fit in when standing in a crowd of much taller people.

Technique/exercise instructions

1 Stand barefoot with your feet hip-width apart.
2 While maintaining big toe and heel contact with the floor, increase your overall height by lifting up through your medial longitudinal arch along the inside of your foot.
3 Slowly lower down again.
4 Repeat for the specified number of repetitions.

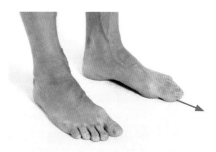

How it should feel It should feel like you are lifting straight up and not just rolling onto the outside of your foot. It's quite difficult to get right, but practice and small, almost unnoticeable movements are fine.

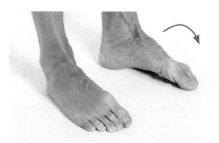

Extra advice Your toes will grab a little on the floor. If you find it easier, do this on a deep carpet.

Equipment (if required) None.

Target area The small and intrinsic muscles of the foot, the lumbricals and the flexor hallucis brevis.

⚠ SAFETY ADVICE/CAUTION

Cramp is the only potential issue here. Ensure you are hydrated and stretch gently if you get some cramp.

PICKING UP MARBLES WITH TOES

BEGINNER: one set of 30 seconds
INTERMEDIATE: two sets of 60 seconds
ADVANCED: four sets of 60 seconds

This is as simple as clearing up a pile of spilled marbles, only using your feet to make them as intelligent and dexterous as your hands. Well… maybe a little closer in ability at least.

Technique/exercise instructions

1 On a carpet or rug, spill some marbles onto the floor.
2 Place a bowl within reach and start to pick up the marbles with your toes and drop them into the bowl.
3 When you've completed the task, change to the other foot and repeat for the specified number of sets.

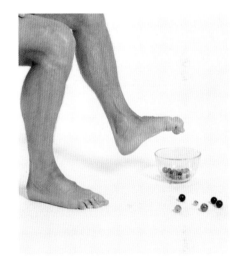

How it should feel Awkward and frustrating, if this is something you need to do. If it feels easy, move on to writing with your toes (*see* p. 156).

Equipment (if required) Carpet or rug, a handful of marbles of different sizes, a bowl.

Target area This works the lumbricals and the flexors of the foot and greatly improves the whole system down there.

Did you know? The hand and the foot have very similar physiology. This means that the foot is capable of almost exactly the same dexterity as the hand, we just detrain it the minute we place our feet in shoes before our first birthday. It's time to undo this lack of training.

⚠ **SAFETY ADVICE/CAUTION** Don't leave any marbles on the floor to be slipped or trodden on at a later stage.

WRITING WITH TOES

BEGINNER: your first name so you can read it
INTERMEDIATE: your full name
ADVANCED: the alphabet

Taking the dexterity of your foot to a whole new level, try holding a pen between your toes and start writing your name. This is the ultimate test for fine movements and micro skill for the foot and toes.

Technique/exercise instructions

1 Tape some paper to a smooth section of floor or onto a flat board or tray.

2 Sit in a chair and place a pen between your toes.

3 Begin writing on the paper with your foot, trying to form a legible version of your first name.

4 Show it to friends and ask them if they can read what it says.

5 Keep on trying until, after weeks of practice, you can write legibly.

How it should feel   Difficult, frustrating and if you are like me, a little stressful – how can something so simple be so difficult?!

Extra advice   You need to spend time doing this and repeating the process to train your brain to restore the fine movements the foot is capable of making. This does not come with rapid rewards and yet is so effective for your long-term running goals.

Equipment (if required)   Tape, paper, a smooth area of floor or a flat board or tray, a pencil.

Target area   The lumbricals and the flexors in the foot.

⚠ **SAFETY ADVICE/CAUTION**   While a felt-tip pen is both a bit wider and a bit easier to control, and makes a mark with less effort, it can have a catastrophic effect on your nice flooring, so be careful with your surroundings and perhaps start with a pencil…

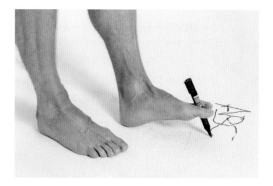

ANKLE

The ankle is the balance and movement manager for the rest of the body. It translates important information to the brain and requires a significant number of muscles, tendons and ligaments to act around it to stabilise and deliver a vast number of movements.

INVERSION STRENGTH WITH EXERCISE BAND

BEGINNER: two sets of 15 repetitions with each foot
INTERMEDIATE: two sets of 20 repetitions with each foot
ADVANCED: three sets of 20 repetitions with each foot

Ankle inversion is the same movement to that which causes a common ankle sprain, in that it is rolling your foot outwards, pivoting along the lateral edge (little toe side).

Technique/exercise instructions

1   Sitting on a chair, loop a resistance band around the inside of your foot, so that the free end is travelling back up the outside of your leg. Take hold of the ends with your hand.
2   Step your free leg over the top of this leg and place your foot in the long section of the band between your outside shin and the band. Push down and away to create tension on the band.
3   To perform the exercise, rotate your foot in and up in an arc, leading with the big toe side of your foot, so you are using the small muscle that runs along the inside of your shin to produce the movement.
4   Slowly release and repeat for the specified number of repetitions.

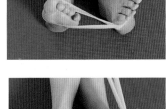

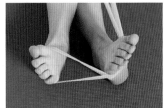

How it should feel   You should feel the muscle on the inside of your shin working, not the muscles on the front of your shin. If this is the case then you are lifting your foot upwards instead of rotating it inwards.

Equipment (if required)   Resistance band of appropriate strength and length.

Target area   Tibialis posterior.

⚠ **SAFETY ADVICE/CAUTION**   These bands can sometimes snap – watch out.

DORSIFLEXION WITH EXERCISE BAND

BEGINNER: two sets of 15 repetitions with each foot
INTERMEDIATE: two sets of 20 repetitions with each foot
ADVANCED: three sets of 20 repetitions with each foot

Dorsiflexion of the ankle is lifting the foot upwards. I remember this by thinking of a dorsal fin on the top of a dolphin, helping me to remember that the dorsal surface is the top.

Technique/exercise instructions

1 Tie a loop of resistance band around a strong table leg or the base of a radiator.
2 Place your foot in the loop, while sitting on the floor with your legs out in front of you and facing the anchor point.
3 Pull your foot up towards you, then slowly return it to the start position.
4 Repeat for the specified number of repetitions on each side.

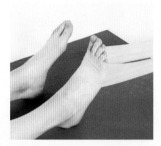

How it should feel   You will feel the muscles on the front of your shin working to bring the foot upwards and then release slowly as you lower under tension.

Equipment (if required)   Resistance band of appropriate strength and length and an anchor point such as a heavy table leg or radiator pipe.

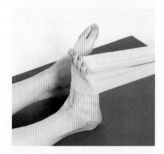

Target area   Tibilialis anterior.

⚠ **SAFETY ADVICE/CAUTION**   If your lower back and hamstring flexibility won't let you sit on the floor with your legs outstretched, consider doing this seated or with slightly bent knees.

> Spread out the band on your foot so it feels more comfortable; it has a habit of bunching up and cutting into the skin after a while.

PLANTAR FLEXION WITH BAND

BEGINNER: two sets of 15 repetitions with each foot
INTERMEDIATE: two sets of 20 repetitions with each foot
ADVANCED: three sets of 20 repetitions with each foot

This is like a calf raise, but using a band. If I'm honest, I like the calf raise more than this exercise, but depending upon your strength and exercise preference this is a good alternative, if slightly more fiddly to set up.

Technique/exercise instructions

1 Start by sitting on the floor with your legs stretched out in front of you. Place the centre of a loop of resistance band around the sole of your foot.
2 Pull the ends of the band with your hands so the band is taut, then push your toes down to work the calf muscles.
3 Return slowly to the start position.
4 Repeat for the specified number of repetitions on each side.

How it should feel Like a calf raise, but potentially a little easier. You can pull harder on the ends of the band to increase the resistance.

Equipment (if required) Resistance band of appropriate strength and length.

Target area Gastrocnemius and soleus.

Did you know? The calf muscle is the only muscle to go through its full range of movement when running.

⚠ **SAFETY ADVICE/CAUTION** Don't let go of the ends of the resistance band – it's like a loaded elastic band being fired.

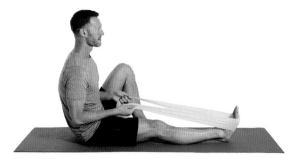
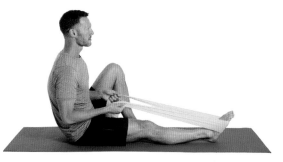

TOE RAISES

BEGINNER: two sets of 15 repetitions on each side
INTERMEDIATE: three sets of 20 repetitions on each side
ADVANCED: three sets of 20 repetitions on each side, plus 20 short-range high pulses on each side

This is a functional version of the dorsiflexion with band exercise on p. 158. It takes the exercise a stage on, since it involves you standing and using gravity as your resistance.

Technique/exercise instructions

1 Stand with your back against a wall.
2 Measure one foot-length distance from the wall and place both feet there.
3 Pivot off your heels and lift your toes as high as you can. Hold for a count of three.
4 Slowly return to the start position. Repeat for the specified number of repetitions.
5 For the advanced setting, at the end of the last rep, lift your toes back up and do some short-range pulses at the top of the movement to finish off.

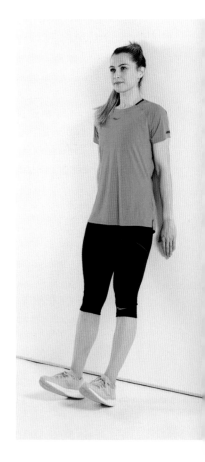

How it should feel   Eventually, you should feel a nice deep burn in your shin area, as you are working the muscles hard. The lateral muscles of the anterior shin are clearly seen working during this exercise.

Equipment (if required)   A wall and some pain tolerance.

Target area   Tibialis anterior

Did you know?   This is a great way to fend off shin splints. Do it nightly and you should be able to dodge this injury.

⚠ **SAFETY ADVICE/CAUTION**   Doing this in socks on a slippery floor can end in a bruised bottom – you have been warned!

LOWER LEG

The lower leg is the driving force for your running speed. Strength here will speed you up, accept ground reaction forces and make you more resilient to injury. What's not to like?

CALF RAISES

BEGINNER: three sets of 15 repetitions on each side
INTERMEDIATE: four sets of 15 repetitions on each side
ADVANCED: five sets of 20 repetitions on each side

Steve Cram used to do 500 of these every day as a young athlete and he broke the world record for the mile more than once.

Even if you don't become a record-holder, the strength gained in the calf muscles will directly and positively affect your running, not to mention reducing injury risk to your calves and Achilles.

Technique/exercise instructions

1 Stand on one leg with your hands against a wall for balance. Lift up on tiptoes and lower down slowly – it's that simple.
2 Repeat for the specified number of repetitions.

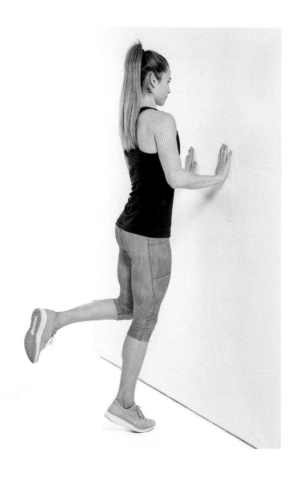

VARIATION: For a much deeper contraction, stand with your toes on the edge of a step and lift up into a calf raise, then slowly lower down until your calves are as low as they can go. Lift back up again. This increases the range and helps to stretch the calf at the same time.

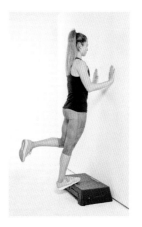 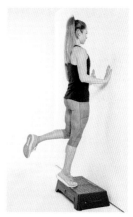

The sets and repetitions shown are great for maintenance, but if you have an Achilles issue follow this protocol:

1 Two weeks of isometric holds for four sets of 45-seconds' duration on alternate days. (Isometric holds for this exercise are standing on tiptoes with no movement at all for the duration of the exercise.)

2 Follow this with six weeks of heavy, slow-resistance calf raises. Follow the action outlined above for the calf raise, but do this slowly up and slowly down for a count of four seconds in each direction. Only do these exercises on alternate days and make them as heavy as possible by loading up a rucksack with some weight.

3 Finish with eccentric calf raises. This requires you to only do the lowering part of the movement with the injured leg. Raise up on your good leg and lower on your injured side as slowly as you can, keeping the speed equal throughout the movement rather than quickly dropping down the first part and only then going slowly, which is what many people do.

How it should feel   Your calf muscles should feel very worked indeed. In fact, it is OK to feel like this exercise has taken your calves to their maximal load in a set of exercises.

Equipment (if required)   None.

Target area   Gastrocnemius and soleus.

Did you know?   There are three main calf muscles. Of these, the soleus is the least known but it is in fact the largest of the three when the medial gastrocnemius and lateral gastrocnemius are considered as individual muscles.

⚠ **SAFETY ADVICE/CAUTION**   Safe as houses.

SHIN STRETCH

BEGINNER: two sets of 20-second holds
INTERMEDIATE: two sets of 40-second holds
ADVANCED: three sets of 60-second holds

This shin stretch is a great one to do after performing the toe raises exercise (*see* p. 160) or if you are suffering with tight or painful shins. The purpose of the exercise is to lengthen the muscles that run along and to the side of the shin bones.

Technique/exercise instructions

1 Kneel down on your mattress or comfortable flooring, or an exercise mat. Sit backwards on to your heels if possible and keep your feet going straight backwards.
2 Sit in the stretch for 20 seconds at first so as not to irritate the anterior shin too much.
3 Repeat for the specified number of sets.

VARIATION: If you cannot manage to go all the way back due to tension in the quads, try doing a quad stretch first (*see* pp. 136–7) or put some pillows under your bottom so you can sit into the stretch.

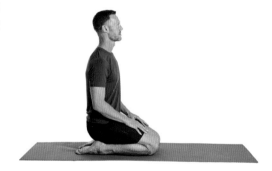

How it should feel   You are aiming for a nice stretch in the front of the shin, but not a harsh pain in the anterior ankle, hence we try to use a soft surface at first.

Extra advice   There is a standing version of the stretch that looks a bit like you are about to kick a ball, but the foot stops on the ground as the toes make contact. You can open up the shin in the same way with good balance but watch you don't fall over or spend all your time wobbling around rather than doing the correct stretch.

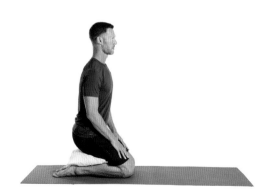

Equipment (if required)   None.

Target area   Tibialis anterior and tibialis posterior.

GASTROCNEMIUS (CALF) STRETCH

BEGINNER: two sets of 30-second holds on each side, daily
INTERMEDIATE: three sets of 45-second holds on each side, daily
ADVANCED: four sets of 60-second holds on each side, daily

The gastrocnemius is the two chicken fillet-shaped muscles in the calf. The medial gastrocnemius is the larger of the two and is on the inside of the leg. The calf is the only muscle that uses its full range of movement when running and is considered one of the prime movers. Stretching the calf is therefore essential. This is one of the most common stretches employed by runners due to its simplicity.

Technique/exercise instructions
SIMPLE STANDING STRETCH:

1 Stand in front of a wall. Place your foot against the wall so the toes are touching it and the heel makes contact with the floor about 7.5cm (3in) from the wall.

2 With a straight leg (locked knee), bring your hip close to the wall until you feel a deep stretch in the calf.

3 Hold for the required length of time without any further movement, then release and repeat for the specified number of sets with each leg.

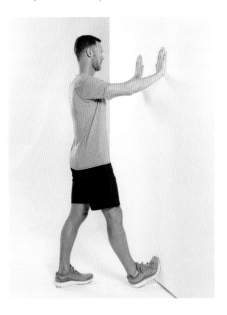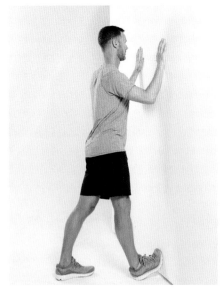

VARIATIONS:

Inversion and eversion calf stretch The previous stretch can be done with the toes rotated inwards or outwards to get a more isolated stretch on either the medial (inside) or lateral (outside) gastrocnemius. Lifting the back heel puts pressure into the correct area and allows you to build the stretch.

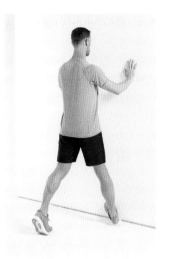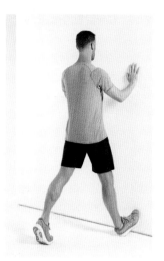

Stretch off a step: The calf stretch can also be done by dropping your heel off a step and lowering into the stretch intensity. This mimics the calf raises from a step, but in this instance it is a stretch and not a strength exercise, so the aim is to lower the heel off a step and then hold for the desired amount of seconds before coming back up, rather than slowly lowering through a wide range of motion.

How it should feel A mild to firm stretch in the location of the calf muscle. This is an easy stretch for most to find and the sensation can be quite intense. If so, ease off the stretch a little and hold in the new position.

Extra advice The calf muscle is vital to stability when running. Wearing heels or a shoe that's raised at the back can chronically shorten the muscle and so if this sounds like you, then make sure you pay additional attention to this stretch and do it more often. And maybe wear more sensible shoes…

Equipment (if required) A wall. Alternatively, you can use a tree, although carrying either of these about is cumbersome and inadvisable…

Target area This stretch will specifically work the gastrocnemius muscles.

⚠ **SAFETY ADVICE/CAUTION** You want to keep this muscle at its optimum length, but once you have the desirable level of ankle dorsiflexion (ability to lift the toes up), then just maintain this. About 45 degrees of dorsiflexion is excellent and should be maintained rather than increased.

UPPER LEG

Have you ever had to walk backwards down your stairs in the morning? After your first race maybe? If you haven't then some would argue that you haven't pushed yourself hard enough yet, but if you have, then you do not need me to motivate you to read this next section.

HAMSTRING STRETCHES 2

BEGINNER: two sets of 30-second holds
INTERMEDIATE: three sets of 45-second holds
ADVANCED: four sets of 60-second holds

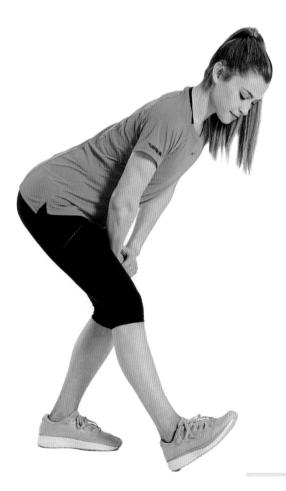

Hamstrings are the bugbear of many, mainly because there are simple tests that everyone does and so they know if they have tight hammies or not and will be quick to tell you just how bad they are. Yet the stretch is so incredibly simple that nobody needs to have to deal with this; it isn't like we're awaiting a cure! We know exactly what to do, it just takes some commitment to the cause and then we can all be more like Jane Fonda. Here are a few more techniques to try out, in addition to the ones on pp. 139–141.

Technique/exercise instructions
STANDING:

1 Place the leg you wish to stretch one reasonable step forwards. Keep that leg straight for now but bend the trailing leg until the knees meet in the middle. Now slightly bend the straight leg, then lean forwards and drop your bottom down a little. You will feel the stretch along the back of the upper leg.
2 Repeat for the specified number of sets.

LYING:

1 Lying flat on your back, take a towel or a resistance band and collect your heel in the central loop, holding the free ends one in each hand.
2 Bring your thigh to 90 degrees to your torso and keep the knee bent.
3 Now pull on the towel or resistance band and your leg will start to straighten. When you feel a good stretch, hold it there for the specified time.
4 You need to maintain the 90-degree bend at your hip, unless your leg can straighten easily, in which case bring the knee closer to you, closing the angle between thigh and torso, then pull the band and foot towards you – so the stretch is always on a bent knee.
5 Repeat for the specified number of sets.

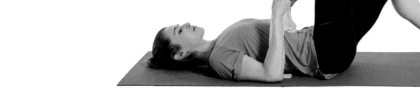

How it should feel The stretch should be felt in the back of the upper leg, where the hamstrings are located. The tendons of the hamstrings cross the back of the knee and insert into the lower leg bone (the tibia), but you tend to find that all the stretch sensation is felt at the back of the knee when the leg is kept straight. This is most likely stretching the sciatic nerve and not the muscle belly, which is high up on the back of the upper leg.

Extra advice Always keep the knee bent so you stretch the hamstrings and not the sciatic nerve. I feel that for running at least we have all moved on from the straight-leg, touch-your-toes stretches common during my school days. Of course, that move is very much still done for yoga, Pilates, gymnastics and various other types of exercise, but not here.

Equipment (if required) A towel or resistance band of appropriate strength and length.

Target area Biceps femoris, semitendinosus and semimembranosus.

⚠ **SAFETY ADVICE/CAUTION** Never lean forwards and bounce into a stretch for your hamstrings – it's not going to lengthen them and will put too much pressure on your back. It also activates a stretch reflex reaction, which is going to prevent muscle lengthening.

HAMSTRING STRENGTH

BEGINNER: three sets of 15 repetitions
INTERMEDIATE: three sets of 20 repetitions
ADVANCED: four sets of 25 repetitions

Strengthening the hamstrings is important. The hamstrings, if being used correctly with a reasonably high heel kick at the back, will be getting a decent workout through your running but rarely through their whole muscle range, so they need a little extra work. They often become tight, so pay attention to the stretch section too.

Technique/exercise instructions

STANDING:

A simple hamstring curl can be done in standing position: simply lift your foot up to your backside and slowly lower it. It is difficult to maintain control when lowering the foot from the very top part of this move, so practise the strength in this range as much as possible.

LYING:

1 To take this to the next level, lie flat on the ground and attach a resistance band to your heel and to an anchor point on the same level as you (a heavy table leg, for example).
2 Lift your foot up to your backside, making sure you have adequate tension all through the action, then slowly lower it back down again.
3 Repeat for the specified number of repetitions.

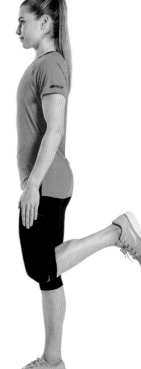

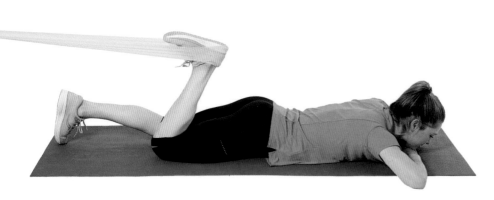

USING A SWISS BALL:

1 This is a great way to strengthen the hamstrings. Lie on your back with your heels on the top of a Swiss ball.

2 Lift your hips up off the ground and pull your heels in towards you using your hamstrings.

3 Slowly push the ball away again. This requires some balance, but is a very functional exercise and worth persevering with until you master it.

4 Repeat for the specified number of repetitions.

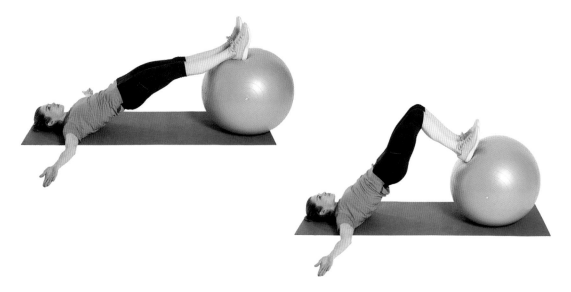

How it should feel The muscle belly of the hamstring is in the back of the upper thigh. This is where you should be feeling the muscle work.

Extra advice Work through the range of exercises until you can manage the Swiss ball workout. It will really improve your running ability.

Equipment (if required) A resistance band of appropriate strength and length and a Swiss ball, widely available online.

Target area Biceps femoris, semimebranosus and semitendinosus.

⚠ **SAFETY ADVICE/CAUTION** The Swiss ball exercise requires some concentration and you have to build up to it. Eventually, you might be able to do it with your arms folded across your chest.

SIDEWAYS SQUATS WITH BAND

BEGINNER: three sets of 10 repetitions on each side
INTERMEDIATE: three sets of 20 repetitions on each side
ADVANCED: three sets of 30 repetitions on each side

This is a combination squat and side lunge. The benefit to you as a runner is that it develops those neglected adductors and abductors in a functional way.

Technique/exercise instructions

1 Tie a resistance band around your legs and spread it out over your thighs.
2 Squat down to a half-squat position (about 45-degree knee bend).
3 Maintain that squat position and step to the side. The band will tighten as you do so, working the abductors of the lead leg. As you slowly lift your trailing leg and step back to the squat, you will also resist the band with your other leg, thus working the abductors eccentrically on that leg.
4 Step to one side for the chosen number of reps, then return to the start position by repeating the exercise, leading with the other leg this time.

How it should feel   Like a crab walking to the side with muscle tension remaining in the quads and glutes for the whole duration of a set.

Extra advice   You can add in some bicep curls when you become proficient, to kill two birds with one stone: developing stronger legs for running and toning your arms at the same time.

Equipment (if required)   A resistance band of appropriate strength and length.

Target area   Abductors and quads mainly, but the whole lower limb is working.

⚠ **SAFETY ADVICE/CAUTION**   Keep an eye on where you are going and hope that onlookers realise that you are doing a training exercise, or else they might think you very strange indeed.

HIP AND GLUTE

The hip and glute form the hinge between the upper and lower body. They are vital to running technique, speed, power and endurance. The muscles of the hip and glute are in almost complete control of the knee and are working tirelessly on posture and forward motion, all at the same time. Respect and look after this key body area as best you can. To find out how, read on.

CLAM

BEGINNER: two sets of 15 repetitions with each leg, daily
INTERMEDIATE: four sets of 20 repetitions with each leg, daily
ADVANCED: unlimited, daily

The clam is a Pilates-based exercise that, when done correctly, works the small glute muscles and in turn aids the control of your knee when running.

Technique/exercise instructions

1 Lie on your side, preferably on an exercise mat or another firm but not hard surface. Bend your knees so that the soles of your feet are in a line with your back. Bend your lower elbow so that you can rest your head in your hand, and place the other hand in front of you for balance.
2 Keep your feet together and lift the top knee upwards, while maintaining your hip alignment. Work hard to resist your hips rolling backwards to gain more movement; it's better to have less movement with a strict exercise.
3 Roll onto the other side to perform the exercise with the other leg.

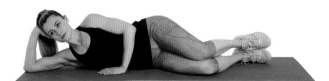

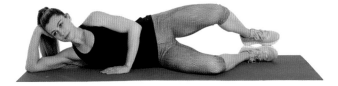

VARIATION:

1 To advance the exercise, get into the start position with your knees bent and heels together, then lift both legs up into the air.
2 Lift up the top leg, as per the clam on the previous page (keeping the feet together).
3 Bring the lower leg up to meet the top knee.
4 Lower the bottom leg again, but keep it suspended in the air.
5 Lower the top leg to meet the lower leg, then lower both down to the ground again.
6 Repeat for the specified number of repetitions, then roll onto the other side and work the other leg.

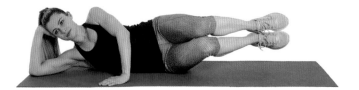

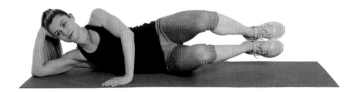

How it should feel   You will feel the small glute muscles working hard after a few repetitions. Keep pushing through the discomfort until you have completed the specified number of repetitions.

Extra advice   You can do this as much as you like – the more the merrier. Your knees will be eternally grateful. The clam is different to the hip abduction exercise on the opposite page in that it works more on hip rotation than pure abduction, but the two together offer the greatest results for your knee control.

Equipment (if required)   Exercise mat.

Target area   Gluteus medius and gluteus minimus.

⚠ **SAFETY ADVICE/CAUTION**   The deep burning pain can be due to ischemic pain, which is a lack of blood flow to the muscle. A few seconds' rest will resolve this and allow you to continue.

HIP ABDUCTION

BEGINNER: two sets of 15 repetitions with each leg, daily
INTERMEDIATE: three sets of 20 repetitions with each leg, daily
ADVANCED: four sets of 20 repetitions with each leg, daily

The knee is controlled by muscles surrounding the hip. This exercise is the first line of defence for knee pain since it will reduce unwanted movement around the knee, reduce pressure on the ankle and inevitably help you to run faster for longer.

Technique/exercise instructions

1 Lie on your side, preferably on an exercise mat or another firm but not hard surface. Bend your bottom knee for improved balance. Ensure that the side of your hip is pointing directly up to the ceiling.

2 Lift your top leg upwards, like opening scissors, to about 45 degrees. Slowly lower down.

3 Before your feet touch, lift up again so the side glute muscles are under constant contraction.

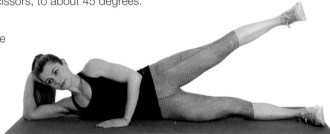

4 Repeat for the specified number of repetitions, then roll onto the other side and work the other leg.

How it should feel   This should start to burn on the area just behind your lateral hip, into the most lateral of the glute muscles. If you are feeling it more in the front of the hip then you have let your posture slide and you are working the hip flexors. Just reset your hip so it's pointing towards the ceiling again and concentrate on keeping it there throughout the movement.

Equipment (if required)   Exercise mat.

Target area   Gluteus minimus and gluteus medius.

⚠ **SAFETY ADVICE/CAUTION**   If you start to get a very constant burning sensation in the lateral hip, this can be ischemic pain (lack of blood flow), so just rest for a few seconds and start again. If the burning persists then it is probably fatigue, so well done, you are working hard!

GLUTE STRETCH

BEGINNER: two sets of 30-second holds on each side, daily
INTERMEDIATE: three sets of 45-second holds on each side, daily
ADVANCED: three sets of 60-second holds on each side, daily

The glute is that thing you sit on all day. The more you sit, the more it becomes long, weak and stupid. The glute activation exercise (*see* p. 70) and this stretch should become two of the most important components of your training if you want to become a faster, less injury-prone runner.

(*see* p. 70)

This is because having a lazy, overstretched and weak glute is going to ensure that you run slowly, put a lot of extra strain on your hamstrings and overload the other muscles in the chain. When we stretch the glute it is not because we have lengthened it through sitting, but because we tighten it in all the wrong places, coupled with lengthening it in all the wrong places. What's needed is balance and equilibrium, so follow the instructions here and you will reap the rewards.

Technique/exercise instructions

1 Lie on your back, preferably on an exercise mat or another firm but not hard surface.
2 Lift the leg on the side you wish to stretch and take hold of the knee with the hand on the same side. Use the other hand to take hold of the ankle and pull the knee and foot towards you.
3 You should be able to bring your lower leg towards your head with as little angle as possible. The greater the angle between the knee and the foot, the less flexible your glute is.
4 Now you have the stretch in this position, try moving the position of the knee more medially and see if the feeling of the stretch changes position or intensity.
5 Keep moving and then holding the stretch in the new position until you feel like all the muscles have had some input from you.
6 Repeat for the specified number of sets.

VARIATION: You can do this in a seated position as well: just perform the same stretch from a chair while at work.

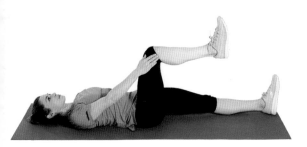
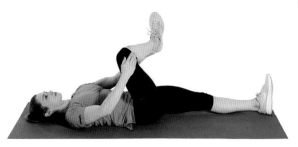

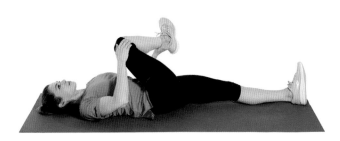

How it should feel   The stretch will feel quite intense and very localised. Hold and move, hold and move, that's the best way to describe this. Always find the greatest stretch and spend at least 30 seconds there. Every day you will feel different levels of intensity in different stretch positions and it is important to keep finding the tightest position and working on that. Within a few weeks the glutes will be in great shape, but always make sure you are strengthening at the same time because we need strength as much, if not more, than flexibility.

Extra advice   The glute is the main hip extensor and therefore the strongest muscle for propelling you forwards. If you don't have a well-functioning glute, your hamstring will take over, tighten and there will be a high chance of some back pain.

Equipment (if required)   Exercise mat and a chair if you do the variation.

Target area   Gluteus maximus, gluteus minimus, gluteus medius and piriformis.

⚠ **SAFETY ADVICE/CAUTION**   If you stretch the same position every time you perform this, you will do as much harm to your running as you would if you simply didn't bother at all. That is why I hate the standard stretch that everyone does as it keeps you in the same position all the time and just lengthens one muscle and leaves all the other muscles tight, causing imbalance.

GLUTE ACTIVATION

BEGINNER: three sets of five repetitions with each leg
INTERMEDIATE: five sets of five repetitions with each leg
ADVANCED: five sets of 10 repetitions with each leg

The glute often does its job of hip extension very poorly indeed, becoming lazy and overstretched through the amount of time we spend sitting down. This exercise will ignite those glutes and change them forever. That's right: you have to imagine you are balancing a tray of champagne on the sole of your foot and then try not to spill any.

Technique/exercise instructions

1 Lie on your stomach on a firm surface. You may want to use an exercise mat. Bend one knee to 90 degrees.
2 Make sure your foot is flat; imagine you have a tray of champagne balanced on top of your foot.
3 Now lift your leg up about 5cm (2in) and slowly lower it down again without spilling a drop of imaginary champagne.
4 Repeat for the specified number of repetitions, then repeat with the other leg.

How it should feel   Your glute should feel like it springs into action and becomes the primary hip extensor. By bending the knee to 90 degrees, you shorten the hamstring too much so it finds it difficult to take over.

Extra advice   Once the glute fires properly, you may start to notice that it fatigues and the hamstrings begin to take over again. It is therefore important that you make this part of your staple diet of exercises each week to maintain the glute activation and build upon it as your training increases.

Equipment (if required)   Exercise mat. You do not need a tray of champagne – just saying…

Target area   Gluteus maximus.

⚠ **SAFETY ADVICE/CAUTION**   Without the tray of drinks, you can come to no harm.

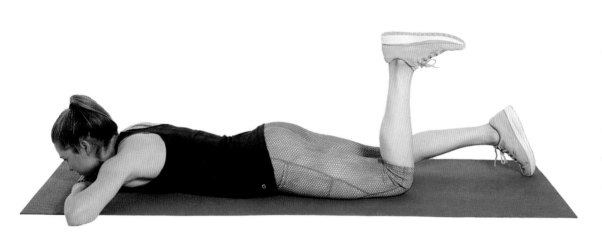

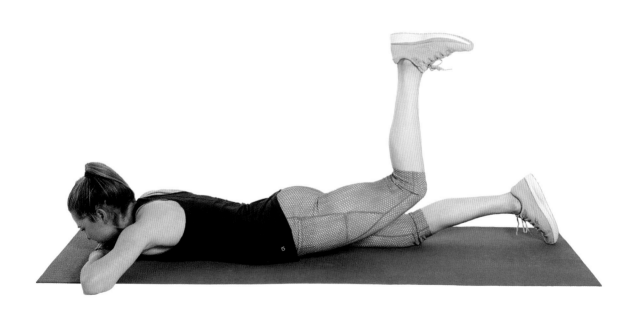

FIGURE 4 PIRIFORMIS

BEGINNER: three sets of five repetitions with three-second holds
INTERMEDIATE: four sets of 10 repetitions with five-second holds
ADVANCED: four sets of 15 repetitions with 10-second holds

Piriformis syndrome (PS) is a potential nightmare. The muscle in the glute lies so close to the sciatic nerve that when it gets too tight, this can cause all the symptoms of sciatica, leaving people reaching for pain medication and an MRI scanner. Left undiagnosed long-term, PS can be tricky to get rid of, especially for the 10 per cent of the population whose sciatic nerve travels through the pirfomis muscle, rather than underneath it. But never fear, use this exercise alongside a good stretch for the glutes and piriformis and you can find yourself cured.

Technique/exercise instructions

1   Lie on your front flat on the floor, head on hands.
2   Take one foot to the back of the knee of the other leg to create the figure 4 position.
3   Now try to keep your hips in contact with the ground and lift your bent knee off the floor.
4   Lift up slowly and try to lower under control. Do the required reps and then swap sides.

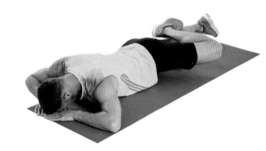

How it should feel   Difficult: you may feel like your knee isn't leaving the floor at all. Rest assured that the instigation of the movement alone is sufficient at first.

Extra advice   The key to this exercise is that only the piriformis works, not the whole glute, lower back, pelvis, etc. So keep those hips in contact with the ground.

Equipment (if required)   None.

Target area   Piriformis.

⚠ SAFETY ADVICE/CAUTION

Try not to extend your back up too much during this; if you do, you will lock your hip flexors out and extend your lumbar spine, making the whole thing more difficult.

HEEL SQUEEZE FOR PIRIFORMIS

BEGINNER: three sets of five repetitions with three-second holds
INTERMEDIATE: four sets of 10 repetitions with five-second holds
ADVANCED: four sets of 15 repetitions with 10-second holds

As you will now know, piriformis syndrome can be at times a disaster. This heel squeeze for piriformis exercise alongside a good stretch for the glutes and piriformis can pay dividends, helping to avoid the onset of PS, and speeding your recovery if you have it.

Technique/exercise instructions

1 Lie on your front flat on the floor.
2 Bend both knees, place the insides of your feet together and spread your knees apart.
3 Now try to keep your hips in contact with the ground and lift both knees off the floor.
4 Lift up slowly and try to lower under control for the required number of repetitions.

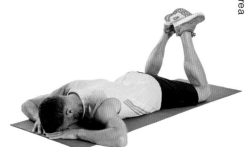

How it should feel   This exercise shouldn't feel like you are doing a form of back extension. You need to leave the upper body relaxed, work from the glutes and lift consciously from them both equally.

Extra advice   As with the previous exercise, the key to this exercise is that the piriformis is working and not the whole glute, lower back, pelvis, etc. Practise this by applying more squeeze to the inner foot to engage the piriformis more than the other glutes.

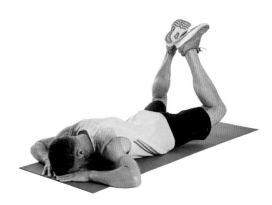

Equipment (if required) None.

Target area Piriformis.

⚠ **SAFETY ADVICE/CAUTION**   This exercise looks so strange, perhaps don't get caught doing it at the office.

SINGLE-LEG SQUAT

BEGINNER: mini squats – three sets of 25 repetitions with each leg, daily
INTERMEDIATE: half squats to full – four sets of 25 repetitions with each leg, daily
ADVANCED: full squats – six sets of 25 repetitions with each leg, daily

The single-leg squat is by far THE BEST exercise for runners. It is the bedrock of just about everything you need, from ankle and foot balance, knee strength and positioning to hip strength and control, with a bit of core thrown in for good measure.

Technique/exercise instructions

1 Stand facing a full-length mirror.
2 Place your fingers on the front of your hip/pelvis area (the nobbly bones at the front of body at belt height). This is so you can watch that you do not drop on the hip as you squat down and that both sides remain level.
3 Start by bringing one foot up behind you, bending at the knee so you are balancing on one leg.
4 Now squat down a small amount by bending the support leg. Watch the knee to make sure you only lower down as far as you can keep your knee in the middle line and over the middle toe. Also, make sure you do not bend so the knee goes over the end of your foot. When your knee starts to deviate inwards come back up and only squat to the depth of this range so that you maintain control.

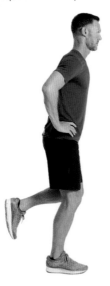 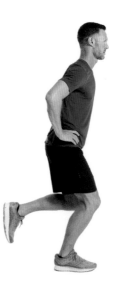

5 The point of this exercise is to only squat to the level at which you retain control and therefore build strength in that range before progressing lower. Each week, try to develop the depth of the squat.

6 Repeat for the specified number of repetitions.

How it should feel The exercise should feel like a combination of balance work and a squat in equal measure. The squat component is strengthening balance. It works on the kinetic chain used during running, builds control of the knee via the muscles at the hip and improves balance at the foot and ankle.

Equipment (if required) Full-length mirror.

⚠ **SAFETY ADVICE/CAUTION** Don't be tempted to go so low that you lose control: all you do is promote faulty movement patterns and make your biomechanics worse.

A lot of concentration is required when you are starting out on your single-leg squat journey. The focus is the knee position and preventing it from moving medially as you squat down. From time to time check the hips, the balance and the like.

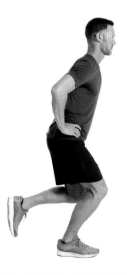 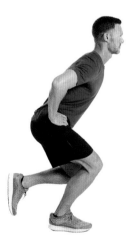

DOUBLE-LEG SQUAT

BEGINNER: three sets of 15 repetitions
INTERMEDIATE: four sets of 20 repetitions
ADVANCED: four sets of 25 repetitions with weight

The squat (called 'double-leg squat' here merely to differentiate it from the single-leg and other types of squat) is a great leg-strength exercise. The glutes and quads are very much in control of this movement and there is no doubt in my mind that you will become a better runner for including these in your exercise diet.

Technique/exercise instructions

1 Stand with your feet shoulder-width apart, toes pointing very slightly outwards if that's the way your knees track naturally.

2 Squat down, taking your arms out horizontally to the side. When you do so, think more as though you are sitting into a seat rather than trying to just get your bottom lower as this will limit the amount you lean forwards. Try to keep your body upright to a degree, although there is a small amount of forward lean required to keep you balanced.

3 Your knees shouldn't pass the ends of your toes as you go down and they should not draw in closer together, or for that matter separate a great deal; try to hold them over the line of the middle toe.

4 Repeat for the specified number of repetitions.

How it should feel Like you are sitting in an imaginary chair, with control through the glutes and quads. The latter have a tendency to burn deep in the muscle once you get going with your repetitions.

Equipment (if required) A mirror is useful. As you graduate through to intermediate and advanced level, then adding hand weights (or wearing a heavy rucksack) is a good idea.

Target area All the quad muscles and the glutes.

Did you know? There are four quadriceps (the clue is in the name). The central one is called rectus femoris, the outside or lateral quad is called vastus lateralis, the inside or medial one is vastus medialis and there is a fourth that lies below vastus medialis and rectus femoris called vastus intermedius. All of these converge into one tendon, which engulfs the knee cap (patella) and then attaches to the top of the shin bone.

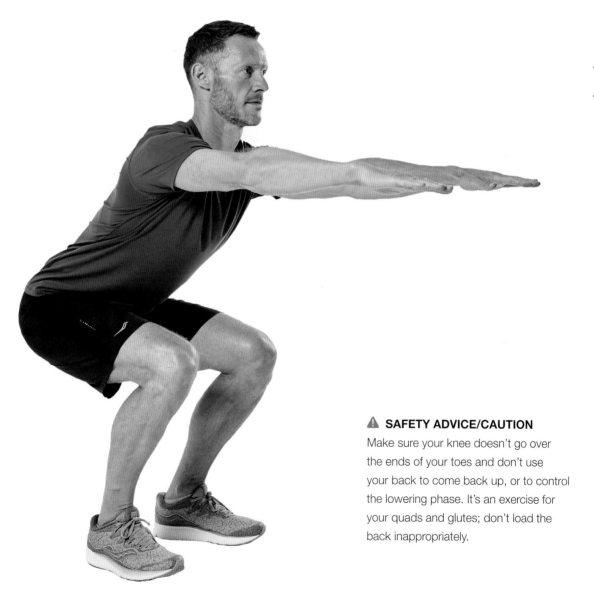

⚠ SAFETY ADVICE/CAUTION

Make sure your knee doesn't go over the ends of your toes and don't use your back to come back up, or to control the lowering phase. It's an exercise for your quads and glutes; don't load the back inappropriately.

CORE

What is the core? Too many people think that the core is the six-pack, but in fact the core is as it sounds: the deep central core of muscles that surround and support your lumbar spine.

To work these, you can't just do a few sit-ups or plank exercises; you need to first make sure you are activating the whole core, then these exercises will work. Want to learn how? Read on.

TA ACTIVATION WITH THREE KEY VARIATIONS

BEGINNER: two sets of 10 repetitions
INTERMEDIATE: three sets of 15 repetitions
ADVANCED: four sets of 25 repetitions

Activating the core largely comes from learning how to activate the transverse abdominus (TA). There is a three-step process for finding your core and a multitude of variations of the exercise that follow once you have achieved true core activation. This is the method that *doesn't* involve using a blood pressure cuff, as you do when you perform a core test (*see* p. 68–9).

Technique/exercise instructions
Finding your core is as simple as 1, 2, 3, core.
1   Lie on your back with your knees bent, like the start position for a basic sit-up. Place your hands on the two little knobly bones of your pelvis, about 5cm (2in) lower than your belly button and on each side of the abdomen.
2   Slide your fingers down a few centimetres and inwards about the same distance. Cough to see if the muscles bounce under your fingers. If not, adjust until you find the right spot.
3   Now you need to activate your core. You do this by following these three simple steps. When all three are happening simultaneously, you have achieved core activation:
   I. Imagine you are going to the toilet and you stop the flow. You will feel the muscles in your lower abdomen on each side tense.
   II. Draw in your belly button towards the spine by using the abdominal muscles and not through breath holding. You can check by holding this for a minute and see if you need to breathe suddenly or simply try talking through the process.
   III. Gently press your lower back towards the floor.

VARIATION 1: Hold your core and at the same time drop one knee at a time out to the side, slowly returning, but holding the core throughout. Repeat for the specified number of repetitions.

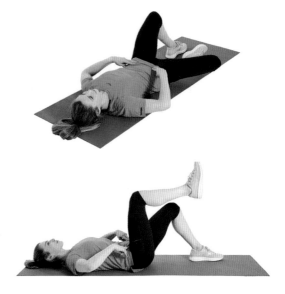

VARIATION 2: Alternate each leg by lifting it up off the floor, while maintaining the same knee bend throughout and holding your core at all times, especially on the direction change and as the leg is placed back down on the floor (the two moments when most people lose control). Repeat for the specified number of repetitions.

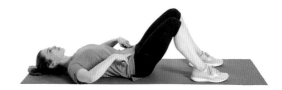

VARIATION 3: Once you have mastered variations 1 and 2, slide your feet further away from your glutes and repeat the exercises, each time increasing this distance for the specified number of repetitions. This will get harder and harder.

How it should feel   You should feel that your muscles are tight and strong around your lower spine and yet you should also be able to breathe easily and hold a conversation. If not, you are simply breathing in and locking your core with your diaphragm during a breath hold, which doesn't help, I'm afraid. Restart the process and try again.

Equipment (if required)   No equipment is needed, although a blood pressure cuff allows you to assess how you are doing. This test is detailed on pp. 68–9.

Target area   Transverse abdominus, rectus abdominus, multifidus, thoracolumbar fascia and internal obliques.

⚠ **SAFETY ADVICE/CAUTION**   Please ensure you do this correctly, every time. Failure to do so 100 per cent properly just means you are giving faulty messages to the core and development is nearly impossible.

BRIDGE

BEGINNER: two sets of 15-second holds
INTERMEDIATE: three sets of 20-second holds with alternating leg lifts
ADVANCED: three sets of 40-second holds with alternating leg lifts

The bridge is a brilliant core-based exercise, utilising the deep core, the glutes and working the lower limbs isometrically. It's a fantastic way of developing your running that offers so much considering how it easy it is to perform.

Technique/exercise instructions

1 Lie on your back on a firm surface, perhaps an exercise mat, with your knees bent and feet flat on the floor.
2 Lift up your hips so they are in line with your knees and shoulders. Make sure the hips do not sag at all. Repeat for the specified number of repetitions.

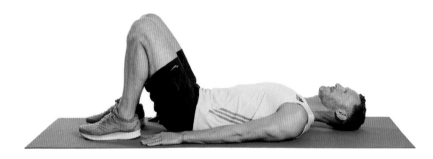

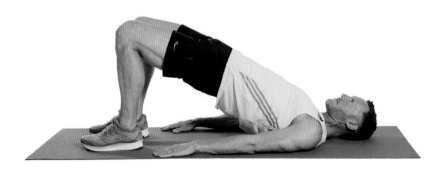

VARIATION: As you become proficient, start lifting one foot at a time, so the hips stay in line but the knee is over the hip. Eventually you may be able to straighten the leg. (*See also* bridge with single-leg lift on pp. 66–7.)

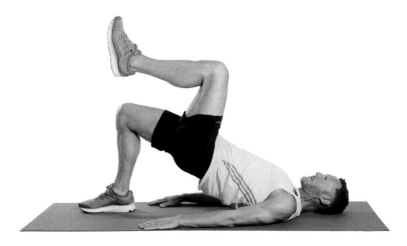

How it should feel You'll feel this in the glutes and the stomach muscles, but you must not give in; maintain the hips at a good level position all in line with the shoulders and knees.

Extra advice The bridge offers a few variations, but largely speaking, bringing your arms closer to your body makes the exercise so much harder. Work yourself through the stages until you can fold your arms across your chest and perform leg lifts. When you can do this, you will be in great shape.

Equipment (if required) Exercise mat.

Target area Glutes, lower back, core, hamstrings.

⚠ **SAFETY ADVICE/CAUTION** This exercise is simple with arms outstretched to the side but loss of balance is possible with the arms close into the body or folded on the chest.

> Without a strong core it is difficult to utilise the strength you possess elsewhere, so build your core first before moving on to leg and arm strength as you will get faster results that are also functional.

BACK EXTENSION

BEGINNER: three sets of 25 repetitions
INTERMEDIATE: four sets of 25 repetitions
ADVANCED: four sets of 50 repetitions

The back extension is a lifting of the head and shoulders from the floor when lying face down, which works the lower back. It is called many things, from the dorsal raise to the McKenzie extension.

Technique/exercise instructions

1 Lie on your front on a firm surface, perhaps on an exercise mat, with your face pointing down and arms to your sides. Relax your legs – they won't be needed.
2 Lift up your head and shoulders from the floor but keep your neck steady by focusing on the floor as you rise up. Do not lift your legs at the same time.
3 Lower back down slowly and repeat for the specified number of repetitions.

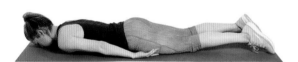

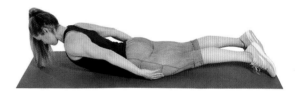

VARIATIONS: As you develop, you can move your arms into different positions to make the exercise harder, with hands above your head or in a crucifix being the hardest as the resistance increases.

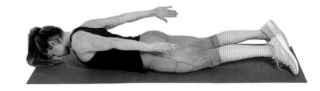

You can also make this more functional by lying on a Swiss ball, with your feet spread at first, but advance as you bring them closer together. The ball needs to be well pumped up so you don't just sink into it and it must be around the lower ribs or stomach for you to be able to perform a good back extension.

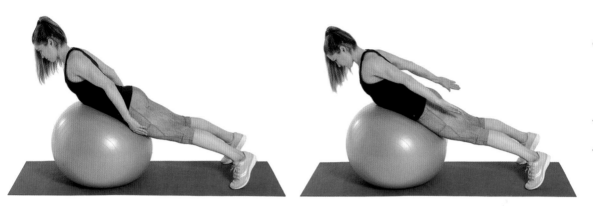

How it should feel You should feel the muscles in the lower back working well. Try not to engage the hamstrings too much as these will want to take over some of the work, which is counterproductive.

Equipment (if required) Exercise mat.

Target area Lumbar spine and glutes.

Did you know? The back extension was the first ever exercise I was given as a young athlete. I still do it today to protect and strengthen my lower back.

⚠ **SAFETY ADVICE/CAUTION** The main safety advice I can give you is to make sure you do this exercise: you are less safe without it in your life.

> Don't forget to engage the core when working the lower back. The core and the back need to learn to work in unison.

SIMPLE SIT-UP

BEGINNER: two sets of 15 repetitions
INTERMEDIATE: three sets of 25 repetitions
ADVANCED: four sets of 50 repetitions

The original stomach exercise, the sit-up, has been the bedrock of all core workouts for decades. Its limitations if used alone are well known, but it still has a place in our training plan.

Technique/exercise instructions

1   Lie on your back on an exercise mat, knees bent and feet flat on the floor (not under anything or being held, since this means it just becomes a poor hip flexor exercise). Place your hands on your thighs.
2   Tilt your chin down ever so slightly to lift the head off the floor and stabilise the neck muscles into a little flexion.
3   Slowly slide your hands up your thighs and to the knees and then back down again. Repeat for the specified number of repetitions.
4   Make the exercise harder by placing your hands by your ear lobes so you have to lift the extra weight of your arms. Stick to the same distance of movement.

How it should feel As you start, it should feel manageable, but depending on the strength of your core, after a certain number of repetitions you'll start to feel a deep burning in your abdominal muscles.

Extra advice This exercise has fallen out of favour a little because it only works the rectus abdominus – the six-pack lines. Worse, it doesn't work them in such a way that the rectus abdominus is functional and working with the lower back and the rest of the core. However, when included as part of a series of core-based activities, it becomes a good addition since it really overloads the muscles in a bit of isolation. Just don't ever rely on sit-ups as your sole core workout.

Equipment (if required)   Exercise mat.

Target area   Rectus abdominus.

⚠ **SAFETY ADVICE/CAUTION** I simply want to reiterate here that doing this exercise without any lower back strength or functional core work alongside is a recipe for disaster. You simply overwork the flexors, which could in extreme cases leave the lower back vulnerable and lead to a stooped posture.

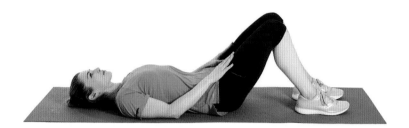

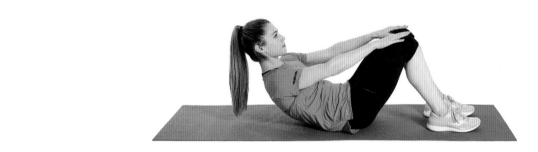

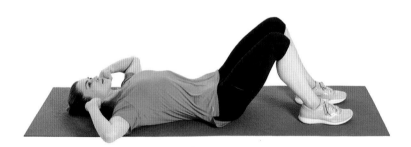

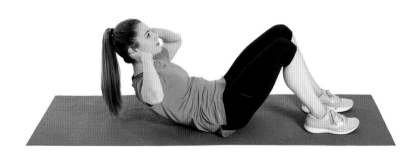

CRUNCH ON BALL

BEGINNER: two sets of 10 repetitions
INTERMEDIATE: three sets of 20 repetitions
ADVANCED: four sets of 30 repetitions

The basic sit-up lacks functional benefits and coactivation of the core and surrounding muscles. However, do the same thing with a Swiss ball under your shoulders and it becomes an incredible exercise.

Technique/exercise instructions

1 Place a Swiss ball between your shoulder blades and then have your shoulders, hips and knees in a straight line with your knees bent to 90 degrees and feet planted firmly on the floor about shoulder-width apart.
2 Fold your arms across your chest and sit up, at the same time keeping your hips level with your knees and shoulders.
3 Slowly lower yourself back down again, keeping control of your pelvis. Repeat for the specified number of repetitions.

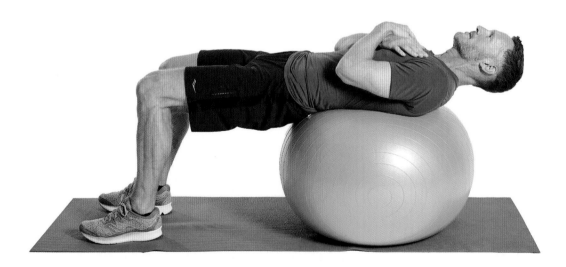

How it should feel Similar to the basic sit-up, this exercise will cause the abdominals to start to burn, but you will also feel the glutes, hamstrings, calf muscles and hip flexors all working along with your lower back. The difference in sensation is clear: you are now working a whole host of muscles together in unison.

Extra advice Balance is a potential issue. Try having your feet wider apart in the early, less-experienced weeks and, as you get stronger, bring them closer together.

Equipment (if required) Swiss ball.

Target area Rectus abdominus, obliques, glutes, hamstrings, lower back, hip flexors and calf muscles.

⚠ **SAFETY ADVICE/CAUTION** Don't fall off.

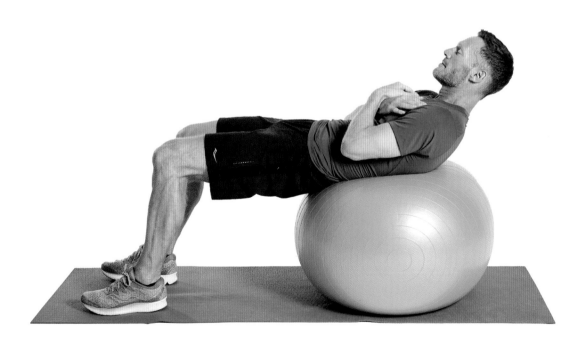

SWISS BALL ROLL-OUTS

BEGINNER: two sets of 10 repetitions
INTERMEDIATE: three sets of 15 repetitions
ADVANCED: three sets of 20 repetitions

For me, this is the ultimate core exercise. It involves everything in one and is very hard to do correctly. I think of this as an advanced exercise, but many think it's easy – it may seem that way to them, but they may well not be doing it right. Done correctly, it takes on a whole new meaning! The challenge is yours to take.

Technique/exercise instructions

1 Start on all fours, then place your hands and forearms onto a Swiss ball on the closest slanting edge. Your forearms will be pointing upwards slightly but you will have control and downward pressure on the ball.

2 Move forwards by pushing your arms along the ball and slowly dropping your hips towards the ground. You need to have 100 per cent control as you do this, so you have an engaged core and do not drop below the straight line you create from head to glute, and through to the backs of the knees, when you are able to get to full extension. Return back up to the start (this is the hardest part if you have gone all the way).

3 If your hands and forearms are in the right place you will not run out of ball surface, so adjust as necessary to allow the full movement.

How it should feel   It's difficult. The slow lowering should feel controlled and balanced – on the way down the challenge is to control several sets of muscles at once – then the route back up should be full of hard work as you contract to close the gap between knees and torso.

Equipment (if required)   Swiss ball.

Target area   Lower back extensors, deep core, rectus abdominus, hip flexors, hamstrings, and stabilisers through the shoulders, neck and upper back.

⚠ **SAFETY ADVICE/CAUTION**

Do not try to push this too hard too early. It is a tricky exercise to get right and so I suggest you start with half repetitions initially.

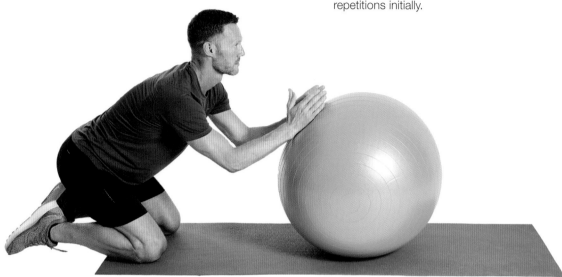

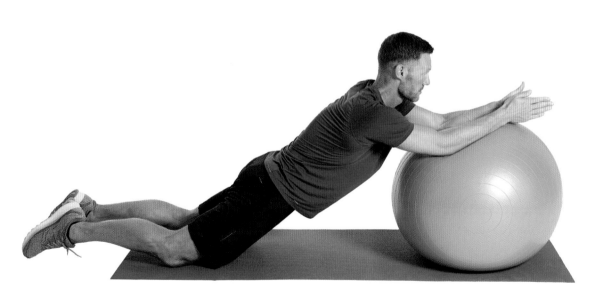

PLANK

BEGINNER: one set of 30-second holds
INTERMEDIATE: three sets of 30-second holds
ADVANCED: three sets of 60-second holds

The plank: the ultimate test of core strength and pain tolerance. Here, the idea is to hold a very rigid low press-up position, with a totally straight body, to utilise your core muscles to prevent any unwanted body movement.

Technique/exercise instructions

1   On an exercise mat, start on all fours, then drop to your elbows and go up onto your tiptoes. Adjust so your back and legs are in a straight line.
2   Hold this plank-like position supported only by your toes and forearms for the specified amount of time and number of sets.

How it should feel   For me it is agony every time, but others love it. The deep core muscles will soon start to shout loudly to your brain to stop, but perseverance is the name of the game, unless of course you cannot hold form, in which case break and try again after a short rest.

Extra advice/tips/did you know?   You can plank from a press-up or on your elbows, the former being more advanced. Always make sure you hold your form. When the hips are sagging it's time to stop; don't work on faulty technique – it's the fastest way to technique faults.

Equipment (if required)   Exercise mat.

Target area   Just about everything gets worked, but the target is the deep core muscles such as the rectus abdominus, multifidus, transverse abdominals and back extensors.

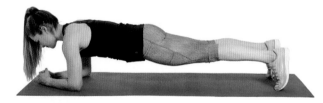

⚠ SAFETY ADVICE/CAUTION

An exercise done well for a short time is worth twice as much as one done badly for any length of time. Check your form is correct.

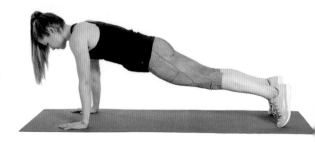

SIDE PLANK

BEGINNER: one set of 20-second holds on each side
INTERMEDIATE: two sets of 30-second holds on each side
ADVANCED: three sets of 60-second holds on each side

The plank, but on your side, supported by your lower foot and the same-side arm. It's wobbly but works the core and side flexors like no other exercise.

Technique/exercise instructions

1 On an exercise mat, lie on your side and then prop up onto your elbow.
2 Lift up your pelvis to align with your shoulders and feet in a slanting line from top to bottom.
3 Hold for the specified time and then relax back down before changing to the other side. Repeat for the specified number of sets.

How it should feel It's like a cross between a balancing act and a sort of gymnastics feat, whereby you balance between your hand or your elbow and your feet. The strain is largely taken in the side of the lower back.

Equipment (if required) Exercise mat.

Target area Quadratus lumborum, internal and external obliques, deep core and hip abductors.

⚠ **SAFETY ADVICE/CAUTION** Make sure you use some sort of mat or your elbow will become irritated.

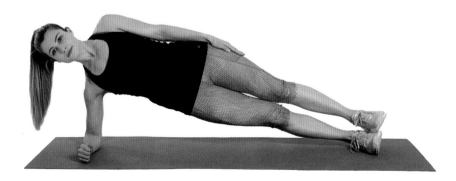

SWISS BALL PLANK

BEGINNER: two sets of 20-second holds
INTERMEDIATE: three sets of 30-second holds
ADVANCED: three sets of 45-second holds

Basically, it's the plank but on a Swiss ball. The addition of the lateral instability makes this a much harder exercise to do properly but more comfortable given that you are at a slight angle and your elbows are on a squidgy, air-filled ball.

Technique/exercise instructions

1 Adopt the plank position (*see* p. 196) with your elbows on a Swiss ball instead of on the floor.
2 Bring your feet closer and closer together until you are being challenged laterally.
3 Ensure that you maintain a straight line through from head to heels with your hips held properly at this exact same height.

How it should feel   You should feel challenged in all directions and be working just as much to maintain stability as you are holding the plank position.

Equipment (if required)   Swiss ball.

Target area   Almost all muscles are being used, but targeted ones are the core, abductors, lumbar side flexors, glutes and shoulder muscles (especially the rotator cuff for balance and control of the shoulder).

Did you know?   Exercises such as this where balance is also a factor work your central nervous system just as hard as the local muscles doing the exercise. The benefits of new neural connections will create a lot of gain for you and your running, so grit your teeth and persevere.

⚠ **SAFETY ADVICE/ CAUTION**
Don't fall off.

ROTATION STRETCH IN SUPINE

BEGINNER: two in each direction, holding for 30 seconds
INTERMEDIATE: three in each direction, holding for 45 seconds
ADVANCED: three in each direction, holding for 1 minute

I usually call this the crossover stretch. It works the lower back but also the whole spine and stretches the glutes. You can't do it standing up, so it's an indoor or dry-grass activity.

Technique/exercise instructions

1   On an exercise mat, set yourself in a crucifix position, lying on your back, legs straight and arms outstretched to the sides.
2   Lift one leg to 90 degrees. Take hold of the now-bent knee with the opposite hand.
3   Pull the knee over your body to the other side and try to get it down towards the ground, while keeping both shoulders flat on the floor.
4   Hold and repeat for the specified time and number of sets.

VARIATION: If you don't have enough rotation flexibility then a shoulder will lift off, the knee won't make it to the ground, or both. If this affects you, try thread the needle (*see* pp. 122–3).

How it should feel   This is a great stretch, felt all along the back but predominantly in the lower back and glute. I think it's the nicest stretch of all and I could literally do it for hours.

Equipment (if required)   Exercise mat.

Target area   Glutes, lower back, thoracic spine, upper back and shoulders.

⚠ SAFETY ADVICE/CAUTION

This isn't safety as such, but sometimes when you're doing this stretch you could feel/hear a popping sound. This is cavitation within your spinal joints and is nothing to worry about at all – it's a normal by-product, which can feel very soothing.

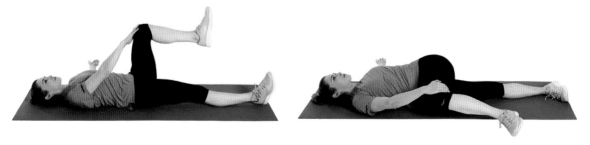

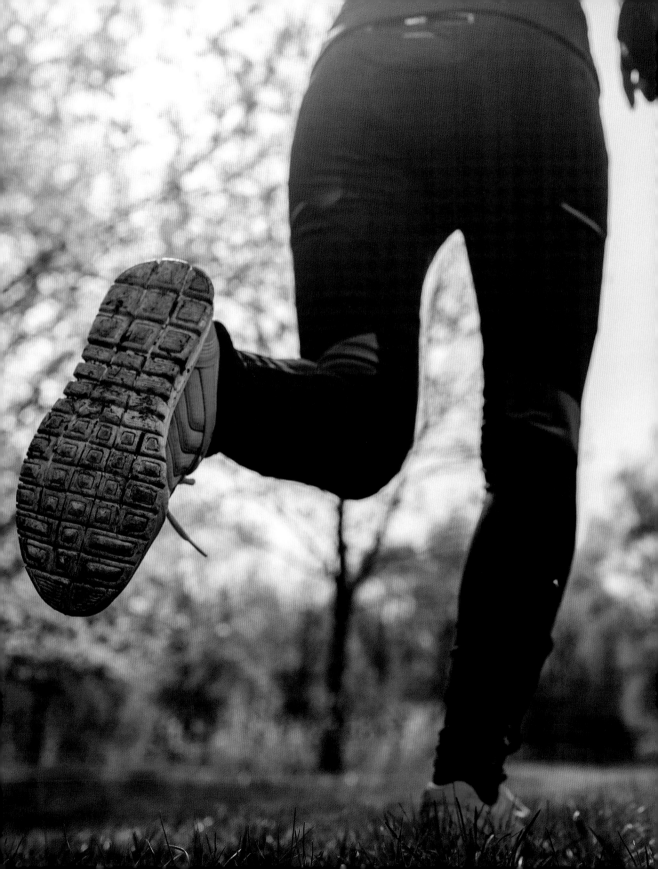

CHAPTER 14

BUILDING STRENGTH

What does it mean to strength train? People become obsessed with strength training and in a way that is great, but you need to understand the basic principles if you are to work effectively and develop your running to its optimal level.

When you provide your muscles with a stimulus that is beyond their normal capacity, they grow stronger on the basis you might try to do the action again and they want to be ready. In short, your body responds to load. If that load then goes away, the body will stop preparing for the extra work and allow detraining to commence. If you always do the same type and intensity of training, the body will simply maintain its level and not fight to grow stronger.

The whole process of training is therefore to keep the stimulus appropriate and fresh; to keep the body guessing and therefore making itself stronger. Simply following a process or exercise because someone once wrote that it was good for your quads doesn't mean anything without a progressive load. For this reason, in this book there is always a progression from beginner to intermediate through to an advanced level.

The fact is, I have no idea what level you are at and so in some cases the prescription offered is an arbitrary guide. You need to learn how to push yourself and to work to the parameters that make the most sense for your own running goals.

I will revisit in the final chapter how best to grow strong for different distances, but in brief: the longer the distance you intend to run, the higher the number of repetitions and the lower the number of sets will be. Those who are trying for a shorter distance will require a greater strength component and need to work at lower repetitions over a higher number of sets.

MULTI-DIRECTIONAL HOPPING

BEGINNER: one set of 30 seconds
INTERMEDIATE: three sets of 30 seconds
ADVANCED: two to three sets of 60 seconds

Once you have mastered the single-leg squat, the box jumps and the plethora of exercises designed to make you a faster, more resilient runner, it's time to step up the challenge somewhat. Welcome to multi-directional hopping.

Technique/exercise instructions

1 Set up some markers. Create a central point from which to start and then arrange a clock face around you, so you have targets to jump for.
2 Starting from the central point, begin at first by hopping to each marker in turn and then hopping backwards to the central point. Change legs and repeat.
3 Now start hopping to random locations in all directions rather than each one in turn.
4 Repeat for the specified number of repetitions.

How it should feel   The hopping should be fun and pain-free, apart from muscle work. You should concentrate on a soft landing each time with a flexed knee and attention to detail when it comes to foot positioning.

Extra advice   Use your arms to increase distance and keep your joints flexed to aid balance, reduce stress and keep the exercise specific to running.

Equipment (if required)   Markers: these could be plastic cones like those used by team sports coaches – anything you can get your hands on that isn't sharp enough to hurt you.

Target area   Glutes, quads, hamstrings, hip flexors, calf muscles and just about every other muscle in the body.

⚠ **SAFETY ADVICE/CAUTION**   We do not want any sprained ankles, so do this exercise on a nice flat surface and make sure you are facing the direction of jump each time and not twisting at any point.

SINGLE-LEG SQUAT ON DECLINE BOARD

BEGINNER: three sets of 15 repetitions, on alternate days
INTERMEDIATE: four sets of 15 repetitions, on alternate days
ADVANCED: four sets of 20 repetitions, on alternate days, with weight

A decline board positions your foot with the toes lower than the heel. Doing the squat in this position really benefits the patella (kneecap) tendon, the quads and your ankle mobility.

Technique/exercise instructions.

1 Stand on one leg on the slope (about 40 degrees is perfect). Place your hands on your hips. Balance and then perform a single-leg squat.

2 Keep the knee over but not beyond the middle toes and maintain balance through the hips. Use your fingertips on the anterior pelvis to guide you as to how level your hips are.

3 Start by squatting down just far enough that you can still maintain your knee position in the central line and then, over the weeks and months that follow, build up the knee bend so you drop lower and lower as control allows.

4 Repeat for the specified number of repetitions.

How it should feel Compared to the single-leg squat, you will notice more loading on the front of the knee. The quads should be felt in use and can burn a bit as you fatigue.

Extra advice There is a latent response, so wait 36–48 hours between sets to allow for collagen synthesis of the soft tissues (*see* p. 37).

Equipment (if required) Slanting board, known as a 'calf stretcher' if you want to buy one. You can also just cut a piece of strong wood to size, preferably not from your dining table – there tend to be complaints about that sort of behaviour…

Target area This exercise targets the quads of course, plus the calf, but its real aim is to strengthen the tendons around the knee – a common site of running injury.

⚠ **SAFETY ADVICE/CAUTION** Wait 36–48 hours between sets to allow for collagen synthesis of the soft tissues, otherwise you may overload them.

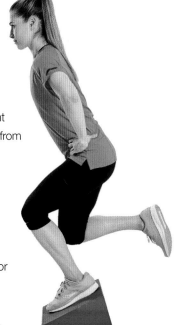

SIDE STEP TO DOUBLE-LEG SQUAT

BEGINNER: two sets of 10 repetitions in each direction
INTERMEDIATE: three sets of 20 repetitions in each direction
ADVANCED: three sets of 30 repetitions in each direction

This is a mixture of the side lunge and the squat. Simply put, you step to the side and squat down, come back up and step to the side again. This is great if you are outside or in a larger space so you can keep working to one side before returning, but if needed you can work in a small space and just alternate the lead leg.

Technique/exercise instructions

1   Rest your arms one on top of the other at chest height. Step to the side and then squat down. Pay attention to the rules of squatting, which are: at all times the knee remains over the middle toe and not beyond, and the hips stay level.
2   Once you have come back up from the squat, bring the trailing leg in.
3   Step with the lead leg again, then drop seamlessly into a squat again.
4   Repeat for the specified number of repetitions on each side.

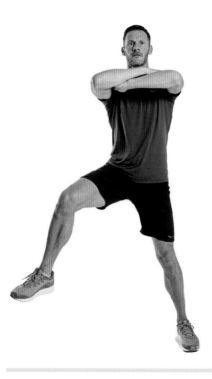
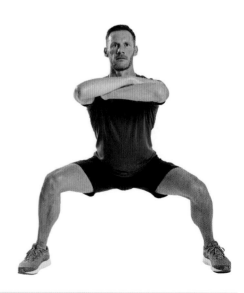

How it should feel This deep lateral squat works the glutes and quads of course but you will also feel it in the adductors along the inner thigh. It's excellent strength work for those races that require more of a lateral movement to get around people who are slower than you are.

Extra advice Once you master the rhythm of the movement, use a resistance band around your thighs to make the side step harder and work the trailing leg more as it has to control the movement inwards between repetitions.

Equipment (if required) Resistance band of appropriate strength and length to go around the legs for the more advanced among you.

Target area Abductors, adductors and quads.

⚠️ **SAFETY ADVICE/CAUTION** No issues at all.

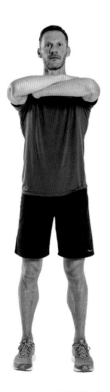

Make sure you concentrate
on the squat when lowering
so you aren't performing
an off-centre squat
with poor form.
Technique is everything.

HIP ADDUCTION

BEGINNER: two sets of 15 repetitions with each leg
INTERMEDIATE: three sets of 20 repetitions with each leg
ADVANCED: four sets of 20 repetitions with each leg

Adduction: the bringing together of the legs. I always think of ADD-uction as being the adding together and AB-duction as taking away – or separating the legs. The adductors are often stronger than the abductors, but we still need to balance ourselves and so some work here is well worth doing.

Technique/exercise instructions

1 Lie on your side on an exercise mat and then bring the foot of the top leg forwards and onto the floor just above the knee of the lower leg, which remains straight.
2 This frees up space behind you for the lower leg to lift up into adduction and then lower back down again.

How it should feel The muscles on the insides of the thighs should feel worked while the rest of the body feels very supported and relaxed.

Equipment (if required) Exercise mat.

Target area Adductor longus, adductor magnus and adductor brevis.

Did you know? This is a staple exercise of the average Pilates class, as are many of the others in this section. If you find the number of exercises overwhelming, consider adding a Pilates session to your weekly routine to do lots of them in one safe hit.

⚠ **SAFETY ADVICE/CAUTION** No issues.

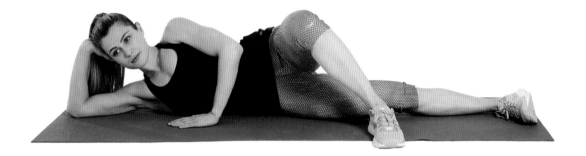

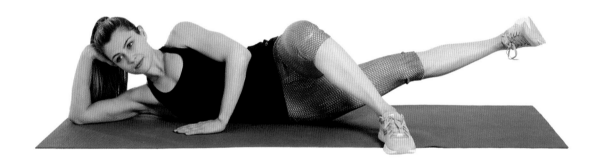

The trick is to keep the pelvis perpendicular to the floor. Use your hand to stabilise your body.

REVERSE LUNGE

BEGINNER: two sets of 15 repetitions with each leg
INTERMEDIATE: three sets of 15 repetitions with each leg
ADVANCED: four sets of 20 repetitions with each leg

The reverse lunge is as simple as doing the lunge backwards in that you simply step backwards instead of forwards. Moving backwards works the muscles in a different way, which is why many technique coaches like athletes to do some backward running to help strengthen the posterior chain. The exercise here is a good compromise and less likely to have you bumping into things and other people.

Technique/exercise instructions

1 From standing, step back and drop your knee to the floor.
2 Step up again and return to standing.
3 Switch legs and repeat for the specified number of repetitions.

How it should feel The emphasis falls to the rear leg, with more work being done with the calf and foot before you load the quads.

Equipment (if required) None.

Target area The glutes, quads, calves and hamstrings.

⚠ **SAFETY ADVICE/CAUTION** Doing this exercise may not be wise for those suffering with plantar fasciitis or ankle sprains as it loads the foot and ankle much more than the forward lunge.

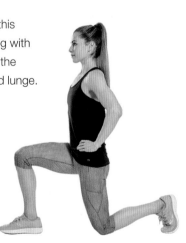
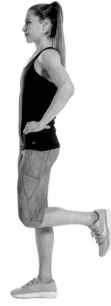

You could combine forward and backward lunges into a nice little mini session for the legs.

DEAD LIFT

BEGINNER: two sets of 10 repetitions
INTERMEDIATE: three sets of 15 repetitions
ADVANCED: three sets of 20 repetitions

The dead lift is one of those age-old exercises that has stood the test of time. Science hasn't found a reason for us all to stop doing it and it seems to bring benefits for the leg and back strength that we so desperately crave.

Technique/exercise instructions

1 Begin by standing with your feet hip-width apart. Soften the knees so they are slightly bent. Hold a 1–2kg kettlebell in your hands.
2 Slowly lower down with a straight back as you slightly bend the knees.
3 Straighten back up again and repeat for the specified number of repetitions.

How it should feel It is hard to keep a straight back, but please try: you want the back extensors to work and also the glutes.

Extra advice Using a kettlebell is great because you can simply aim this between your feet.

Equipment (if required) A weight of some description. This could be a small kettlebell, a large container of water, dumbbells or a barbell (most common).

Target area The dead lift works the hamstrings very well indeed, in addition to the glutes and the lower back.

⚠ **SAFETY ADVICE/CAUTION**
Please do keep your knees soft and slightly bent; the force you otherwise put through your lower back can be damaging.

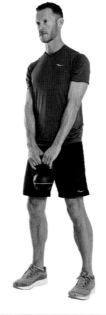
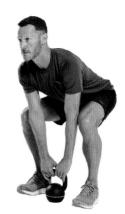

BOSU® WORK: SQUATS AND OVERHEAD PRESS

BEGINNER: two sets of 10 repetitions
INTERMEDIATE: three sets of 15–20 repetitions
ADVANCED: four sets of 20 repetitions

BOSU® stands for 'Both Sides Utilised'. These discs have one flat, inflexible side and one domed, inflated side. Working on a BOSU® is brilliant for training your balance and your core, while at the same time doing some fantastic exercises.

Technique/exercise instructions

THE SQUAT:

1   Position the BOSU® with the round inflated side downwards and the flat plastic side uppermost.
2   Stand on the flat side in a fairly wide stance, ensuring your feet are on equally in all directions to assist balance. You may wish to put your arms out to the front to help you balance.
3   Once you're settled and have your balance, slowly do the first squat.
4   Slowly come back up, giving yourself time to adjust to the extra movement.

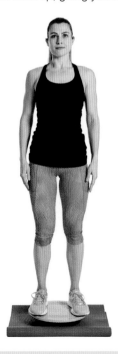
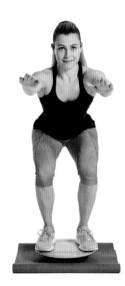

OVERHEAD PRESS:

Once you can do a basic squat you can start to do some other exercises, such as overhead press. If you want to incorporate the bicep curl in every movement then that is slightly more advanced but very good in its own right as an exercise.

1 Stand on the BOSU® as before, this time with a dumbbell in each hand.

2 With your elbows tucked in, bicep curl the weight to shoulder height and then press up above your head.

3 Return the weight back down to your shoulders and repeat.

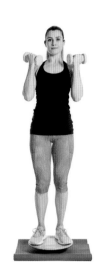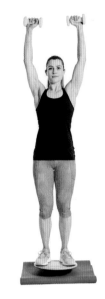

SINGLE-LEG SQUAT:

For the adventurous, you can do some single-leg squats on the BOSU® as well.

1 Simply move one foot to the middle of the BOSU®, get your balance and squat down slowly, maintaining your alignment (*see* pp. 180–1).

2 Slowly return to standing, then repeat.

How it should feel The primary goal here is to test and train balance, but you get to do some other good work at the same time. That said, the overall feeling is one of trying to stay on the BOSU®, training your central nervous system.

Extra advice Although often quite expensive, the BOSU® is a phenomenal piece of equipment.

Equipment (if required) BOSU®.

Target area The whole body.

⚠ **SAFETY ADVICE/CAUTION** You need to be in the right frame of mind to keep your balance when you do this.

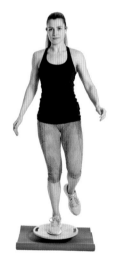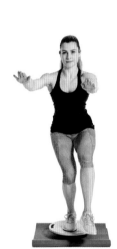

STEP-UP ONTO BOX

BEGINNER: three sets of 10 repetitions with each leg
INTERMEDIATE: three sets of 15 repetitions with each leg
ADVANCED: three sets of 20 repetitions with each leg

Think of this as going up a really big flight of stairs, but each step one at a time. This will maximise your strength in the running motion and make hills feel easy.

Technique/exercise instructions

1   Stand facing a box or step.
2   Step up with one leg, then step down with the other.
3   Repeat the motion so as to load the same leg for the specified number of repetitions, then switch to the other leg.

VARIATION: You can then add weight either by holding dumbbells or by using a barbell across your shoulders.

How it should feel   Like a hard quads and glute workout.

Extra advice   Make sure your knee stays over your middle toes when you step up; a lack of control or too much weight can sometimes cause you to drop your knee into the midline so keep an eye on that and ease off the weight or number of repetitions until you regain control.

Equipment (if required)   A step or box and some weights.

Target area   Primarily the glutes and quads.

⚠ **SAFETY ADVICE/CAUTION**   Keep that knee alignment and ask someone to stand behind you if you start to use heavier weights, in case you slip or fall.

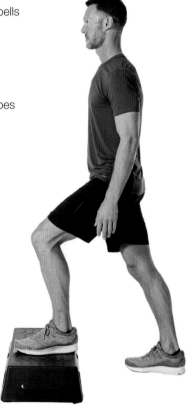

BOX JUMPS

BEGINNER: one set of 10 repetitions
INTERMEDIATE: two sets of 10 repetitions
ADVANCED: two sets of 15 repetitions

This exercise is a demonstration of power and agility as well as explosive strength – it involves jumping double-footed from the floor onto a box.

Technique/exercise instructions

1 Stand facing a box, bend your knees and jump up onto it so that you land with both feet hip-width apart in the middle of the box. Swing your arms to aid the movement.
2 You can then step back down to the start position before repeating the action, or jump down forwards, turn and repeat by jumping up onto the box again.
3 Repeat for the specified number of repetitions.

VARIATION: Alternatively, arrange a row of boxes in a line and jump up onto one then down and up onto the next to make this a plyometric exercise. This exercise is advanced and should only be done by people who are very confident with their squats, squats with weight and step-up onto a box with weight.

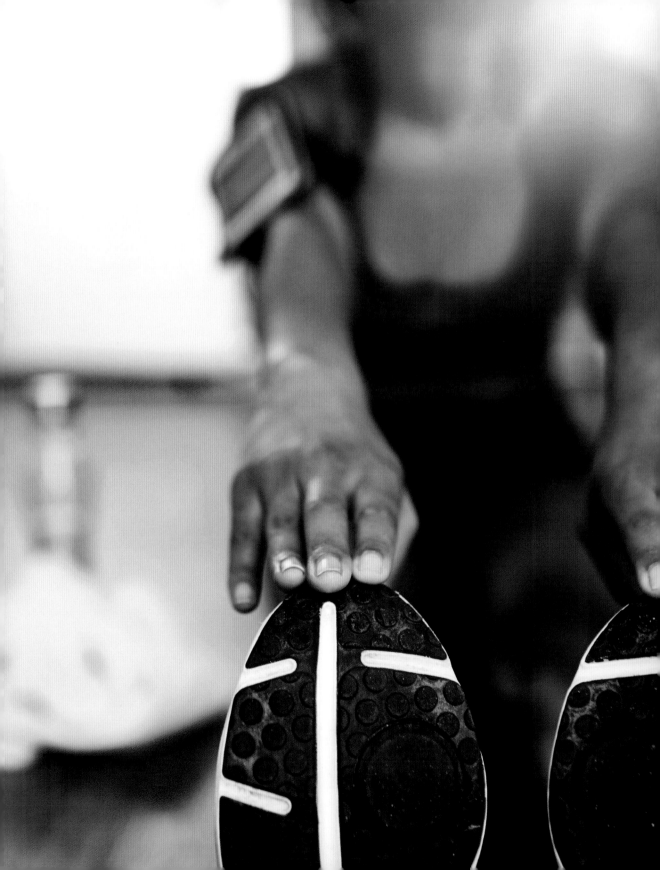

CHAPTER 15

STRENGTH AND CONDITIONING WORKOUTS

Strength and conditioning workouts are a prerequisite for attaining more from your running. Without these in your programme, you are both at risk of injury and, worse, a plateau in your performance.

The principles of training are to produce an overload for the tissues, to make the training specific to your goal and to consider that once a level is reached it needs to be maintained or the effects of the training are reversible. With that in mind, it is important to realise that a sprinter will spend more time lifting very heavy weights compared to the lighter weights lifted more times by a marathon runner. A marathon runner has little need to produce a maximal effort during the course of their race but requires muscle endurance so they can keep producing submaximal work many times over. A strength and conditioning (S&C) workout should fit the needs of the athlete.

This does not, however, take into account significant muscle imbalances and weaknesses that a runner already has, which will need specialist work using specific exercises to restore balance. What follows is a guide to what to do when everything is working well and you are looking for performance gains. If this isn't you, you need to first achieve balance.

Over a year, you have some specific phases of training. Taking the competition phase out of the equation for now, let's look at what happens straight after the season and then work our way back around to the start of the next season.

Up until your final race, say in August or September for most, the body has been utilising the gains made by hard training blocks of pre-competition build-up. However, due to a heavy track season, the ability to keep some of the fundamentals of training going has been compromised. It follows, then, that after a well-earned break for a couple of weeks, you need to revisit the injuries and weaknesses that have piled up over this period and start to address them.

The early period of this training should form a sort of deconstruction of the body – featuring lots of assessment and a review of the year – to tell you what needs most work. For example, ask yourself whether the final third of each race demonstrated a lack of fitness as everyone overtook you, or whether your start was slow and weak and made it much harder for you to get back on terms with the other runners. The answers to these sorts of questions will provide you with the information you need to start to create your new S&C programme for the coming year. Of course, the form this programme takes depends on the type of running you are doing, so let's break it down and assess the different requirements.

TRAINING SET REPETITION		
TRAINING GOAL	REP	WORKING SET
Endurance	12 or more	two to three
Hypertrophy (muscle size)	six to 12	three to six
Strength	six or fewer	two to six
Power	one to two	three to five

STRENGTH FOR SPRINTING

Sprinters will need maximal muscle contraction and at a high speed of turnover. Strength is therefore paramount, but strength without power is going to leave you in the starting blocks while every other athlete is on their way to the finish line.

Pure strength training is seen as very heavy weights lifted from one to six times in a set and usually comprises four or more sets.

Power training is all about the explosive nature of the movement, but again the weights will be heavy and the repetitions even lower, one to two repetitions at a time. For both strength and power, the rest periods will be quite long to allow for local muscle energy to return in the form of adenosine triphosphate (ATP).

You would add into this programme some plyometric training, which is very explosive. This could include sequential box jumps, whereby, for example, you jump up onto a box, then jump down into the space between that box and another higher box, and with minimal contact time bound up onto the next box, and so on. The boxes are often of varying heights.

STRENGTH FOR MIDDLE DISTANCE

Middle-distance runners will still require strength but also a lot of strength endurance with less power. The middle-distance runner needs to be able to produce a high number of sub-maximal contractions, but these sub-maximal contractions are still at a very high level as they are working in the high-energy zones for the duration of the race.

I would say middle-distance runners need to be good at everything – strength, power and endurance – but most of all they need to be able to work at their anaerobic threshold for extended periods of time. The anaerobic threshold is the point at which the blood is accumulating a lot of lactic acid. If someone goes too far beyond this point, they will end up becoming too fatigued and needing to stop.

The ability to utilise strength and aerobic fitness all at once is the product of a very mixed training regime and does not come from just running alone. Three to six sets of six to 30 repetitions would be the range of this sort of S&C programme.

STRENGTH FOR 5/10K

Similar in training requirements to middle-distance events, the 5km is a distance that requires a high capacity for sustained exertion. Slightly lower muscle contraction is required than for middle distance, but only just, and as such the training will not vary too much. There is a reduced need for high muscle strength for 10km races, although more is required than would be needed for a marathon, for instance. Three sets of 15 to 20 repetitions would be the mainstay of this sort of S&C programme.

STRENGTH FOR HALF-MARATHON OR MARATHON

When running a marathon distance you really need endurance, but to avoid all types of strength training would be detrimental to your ability to withstand the loads of training and also the eventual time it takes you to cross the line.

For endurance, I like to recommend very high repetitions, working over total number of repetitions rather than three sets of 12 for example. A good session is to aim for 100 repetitions on each exercise. This could be as simple as four sets of 25 repetitions or you might consider really going for it and doing a maximal count of 50 repetitions until fatigue, then going again after 30 seconds' rest and maybe doing 20 repetitions, then another rest, before managing 12 repetitions, and so on until you have done all 100 repetitions with short rests. This is brutal but great for endurance.

FINAL WORD

You will have been on a journey through this book and sometimes you may have thought the simple exercises didn't actually teach you anything new. However, it's likely that you will have also stumbled across exercises that pushed you and you perhaps even found impossible so here is the point: you have to be able to do the basics well if you want to achieve expert status at the more complex exercises.

We are taught a great deal of exercises badly by a number of people as we develop into athletes. It might be the PE teacher from school, or the gymnastic coach you once had, or the exercise class instructor who didn't much care for the preparation. Over the last decade or two of your fitness journey things have changed and perhaps your faulty technique hasn't been modified by anyone along the way.

It is possible to look at a glute stretch and think, 'Oh, I know that one,' move on and try to find something you haven't seen before. I urge you to go over the basics once more – really check your beliefs against the technique points in this book, try the exercise as if you are doing it for the first time. If you really want to consider yourself an expert at these basic techniques, then try to teach someone else to do it correctly. Teaching others is one of the highest forms of learning.

With all my books (all two of them now) I do try to inject a little humour. This is because at times it can be a dry subject and I want to make sure nobody switches off. If you found anything funny then great, if not then I apologise. Either way, the points I am making are still serious. Just because I reference a side lunge as being similar to a drunk uncle at a wedding dancing with his tie wrapped around his head doesn't mean that the side lunge is not important. I am merely enabling you to have some fun with the exercise and also giving you an easy way of recalling it when needed.

If I could have one wish it would be that this book could in some way be a prequel to my first, *Running Free of Injuries* (*RFOI*), on the basis that you use *RFOI* when you become injured, but this one to offset the chances of becoming injured in the first place. Sat side by side on your bookshelf, I believe they combine to make a user-friendly, one-stop shop for today's runner.

Feedback from *RFOI* was so great and I was delighted that it made number one in the Amazon chart. I was especially happy that people commented that they found it easy to read, many stating that it broke away from the norm of a dry, academic tome and some people saying they read it from cover to cover. This is perfect as it was my absolute aim.

One of the greatest forms of feedback comes when the person giving it doesn't know you are listening. I experienced this one day at a running expo. As I passed the Bloomsbury stand, two young physios were talking and having a bit of a contest with one another. One picked up my book, flicked through and reported to his physio colleague: 'Well, this is a bit basic for me really, but I suppose it would be good for a runner or young physio.'

I love this so much for two reasons: first, I didn't want the book to be an academic chore to read and second, I was once like this young physio, full of my own self-confidence and worth. I am now, by contrast, much more aware of the things I do not know and am very comfortable and actually happy to admit them openly. Everyone goes on a journey, which really has no particular destination except education. Failing to understand what you do not know is the biggest barrier to learning and dismissing something in the vein of 'I already know that' is one clear way to limit your potential.

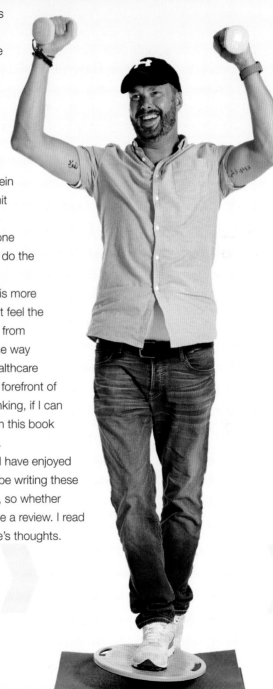

Do the basics well. If this book gives you one vital piece of information, it is that you should do the basics well.

Maybe one day I will write something that is more complex and challenging, but I honestly didn't feel the need to join my two young physio colleagues from that running expo and write this book as some way of showing off to or competing with fellow healthcare practitioners. Instead, I kept the runner in the forefront of my mind as I wrote every word and I kept thinking, if I can just get them doing the basics really well, then this book will have a much greater impact on their lives.

So I hope you enjoy this book, I really do. I have enjoyed writing it so much that I am genuinely sad to be writing these last sentences. I love feedback of all varieties, so whether you liked the book, or hated it, please do write a review. I read them personally and look forward to everyone's thoughts.

Safe running.

Paul

ACKNOWLEDGEMENTS

This book would not have been possible without a vast number of people, but in chronological order... My parents Margaret and John, for without their love and support and gushing pride I would never have amounted to anything. They are my rock and my guiding light and I love them dearly.

For every minute spent writing the book I had to neglect my family, so thank you to my poor wife Nicola, who has been simply amazing throughout, even though she was demented trying to juggle our three amazing, effervescent kids, Harriet, Archie and Brodie. Through the book-writing phase Brodie was just seven years old and would periodically come and ask me if my book was finished yet, mainly because he needed me to attend to his need for an in-bedroom zip wire for his teddies. He put more pressure on me than Bloomsbury ever could or would.

Archie joined me in a creative way by teaching himself the drums during my writing sessions, which was amazing to be part of, but at times... well, you can picture the scene, right? Either way, he is now really quite accomplished and it's amazing to hear.

Harriet, our eldest, joined Archie in the wilful destruction of the required peace and quiet. She is quite the singer. I don't mean just for play, I mean people pay her to sing for them and I suspect by the time this book hits the printers she may well already be known to you. This could be father's pride, so forgive me.

So to my three kids, I burst with pride every day because of you, just keep the chuffing noise down for book three... You are the product of an amazing mother who has dedicated her life to you and me and for that we should all be acknowledging her as the real hero of our achievements. This book is for you, Nicola.

I have to also thank my staff, who have carried the can at work, expertly, accurately and without complaint. Physio&Therapy UK is alive and well because I trust them implicitly and that comes from mutual respect, which I am very proud of indeed.

Lastly to Bloomsbury, the publisher who should be everyone's first choice. Matt, you have been the carrot and the stick and used perfect measures of both throughout. I couldn't thank you enough.

BIBLIOGRAPHY

Fowles, J. R., Sale D. G. and MacDougall J. D. (2000) 'Reduced strength after passive stretch of the human plantarflexors', *Journal of Applied Physiology* 89(3), 1179–1188

Hobrough, P. (2016) *Running Free of Injuries: From Pain to Personal Best* (London: Bloomsbury)

Horowitz, J. (2013) *Quick Strength Training for Runners* (Boulder, Co.: Velo Press)

Jarvis, M. (2013) *Strength and Conditioning for Triathalon: The 4th Discipline* (London: Bloomsbury)

Malanga, G. and DeLisa, J.A. (1998) 'Gait Analysis in the Science of Rehabilitation', U.S. Department of Veteran's Affairs www.rehab.research.va.gov/mono/gait/malanga.pdf [accessed September 2019]

Nelson, A. G., Kokkonen J. and Arnall D. A. (2005) 'Acute Muscle Stretching Inhibits Muscle Strength Endurance Performance', *Journal of Strength and Conditioning Research* 19(2), 338–343

Norris, C. M. (2008) *Stretching for Running* (London: Bloomsbury)

Rolf, C. (2007) *The Sports Injuries Handbook* (London: Bloomsbury)

Seijas Albir, G. (2015) *Anatomy and 100 Stretching Exercises for Runners* (New York: Barron's Educational Series)

Shepherd, J. (2013) *Strength Training for Runners* (London: Bloomsbury)

Thompson, D. (2001) 'Muscle Activity During the Gait Cycle', University of Oklahoma ouhsc.edu/bserdac/dthompso/web/gait/kinetics/mmactsum.htm [accessed September 2019]

www.physio-pedia.com

INDEX

Index of exercises